Forschende
Komplementärmedizin
Wissenschaft • Praxis • Perspektiven

Supplement 1,
Vol. 14,
April 2007

International Congress on Complementary Medicine Research

Munich, May 11–13, 2007

ABSTRACTS

Editors

Dieter Melchart, Munich, Zurich
George Lewith, Southamton
Wolfgang Weidenhammer,
Klaus Linde, Munich

TECHNISCHE UNIVERSITÄT MÜNCHEN

International Society for Complementary Medicine Research

Klinikum rechts der Isar, München

KARGER

Basel · Freiburg · Paris · London · New York ·
Bangalore · Bangkok · Singapore · Tokyo · Sydney

Forschende
Komplementärmedizin
Wissenschaft • Praxis • Perspektiven

Contents

KARGER
Fax +49 761 4 52 07 14
E-mail Information@Karger.de
www.karger.com

Accessible online at:
www.karger.com/fok

print
ISSN 1661–4119
Forsch Komplementärmed
14(S21) VIII+1–56 (2007)
ISBN 978-3-8055-8312-1
14 S1 07
online
ISSN 1661–4127
www.karger.com/fok

Forschende Komplementärmedizin

Wissenschaft • Praxis • Perspektiven

Research in Complementary Medicine

Research • Practice • Perspectives

International Congress on Complementary Medicine Research

Munich, May 11–13, 2007

ABSTRACTS

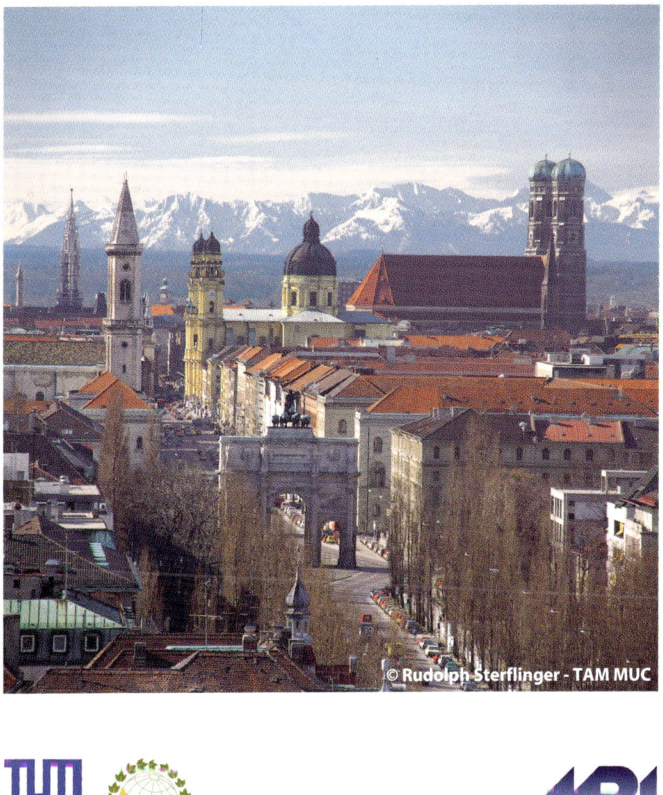

Editors

Dieter Melchart,
Munich, Zurich
George Lewith,
Southamton
Wolfgang Weidenhammer,
Klaus Linde, Munich

S. Karger
Medical and Scientific Publishers
Basel · Freiburg · Paris ·
London · New York ·
Bangalore · Bangkok ·
Singapore · Tokyo · Sydney

KARGER

TECHNISCHE UNIVERSITÄT MÜNCHEN

International Society for Complementary Medicine Research

Klinikum rechts der Isar, München

Band 14, Supplement 1, April 2007

Offizielles Organ der Schweizerischen Medizinischen Gesellschaft für Phytotherapie
Offizielles Organ der European Society for Complementary and Natural Medicine

Forschende Komplementärmedizin

Wissenschaft • Praxis • Perspektiven

Research in Complementary Medicine

Research • Practice • Perspectives

Informationen, Anfragen bitte direkt an:
S. Karger Verlag für Medizin
und Naturwissenschaften GmbH
Dipl. Psych. Franziska Lang
Lörracher Straße 16a
D-79115 Freiburg
f.lang@karger.de

KARGER

Basel · Freiburg · Paris · London · New York ·
Bangalore · Bangkok · Singapore · Tokyo · Sydney

Impressum

Die Zeitschrift erscheint zweimonatlich; pro Jahr erscheint 1 Band zu je 6 Heften. Bezugspreis für Jahrgang 14, 2007: Print-Abonnement EUR 164,–, Online-Abonnement EUR 164,–, Kombi-Abonnement Print/Online EUR 208,–, einschließlich MWSt., zuzüglich Postgebühren. Der Abonnementpreis ist im Voraus zahlbar. Das Abonnement der Zeitschrift läuft weiter, wenn es nicht spätestens 4 Wochen vor Abschluss eines Bandes abbestellt wird. Abonnementbestellungen können bei jeder Buchhandlung oder direkt beim Verlag aufgegeben werden:

Deutschland:
S. Karger Verlag für Medizin und Naturwissenschaften GmbH
Lörracher Str. 16a
D-79115 Freiburg
Tel. +49 761 45 20 70
Fax +49 761 4 52 07 14
E-mail Information@Karger.de

Übrige Länder:
S. Karger AG
Allschwilerstr. 10
Postfach
CH-4009 Basel
Tel. +41 61 3 06 11 11
Fax +41 61 3 06 12 34
E-mail Karger@Karger.ch

Anzeigen:
S. Karger Verlag für Medizin und Naturwissenschaften GmbH
Lörracher Str. 16a
D-79115 Freiburg,
Tel. +49 761 45 20 70
Gültig ist die Preisliste Nr. 10 vom 1. Januar 2007.

Supplement 1 zu Band 14, April 2007
ISBN 978-3-8055-8312-1

Verlagsleitung und presserechtlich verantwortlich: Sibylle Hopf
Produktionsleitung: Georg Brunner
Anzeigenleitung: Susanne Meister

Gesamtherstellung:
KONKORDIA GmbH, Bühl
Das Medienunternehmen

Bibliographische Dienste
Index Medicus/MEDLINE
Current Contents/Clinical Medicine
Science Citation Index Expanded

Titelbild «Nr. 711 Münchner Panorama mit Blick auf die Alpen»
© Rudolph Sterflinger – TAM MUC
Mit freundlicher Genehmigung vom Tourismusamt München

KARGER
Fax +49 761 4 52 07 14
E-mail Information@Karger.de
www.karger.com

© 2007 S. Karger GmbH, Freiburg

Accessible online at:
www.karger.com/fok

Traditional uses and health beneficial effects of selected local food plants

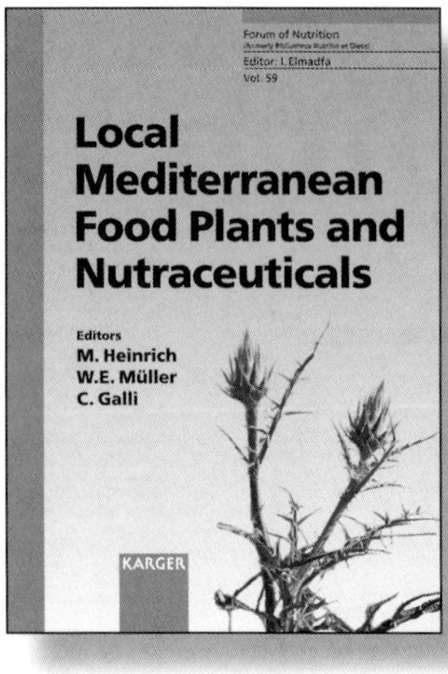

Local Mediterranean Food Plants and Nutraceuticals

Editors
Michael Heinrich
Walter E. Müller
Claudio Galli

Nutrition, Clinical Nutrition, Dietetics, Anthropology, Botany, Micronutrients, Phytomedicine, Pharmacology, Gerontology, Cardiovascular System, Oncology

As a result of domestication – considered to be the most important cultural development of the past 13,000 years of human history - we depend today on a tiny number of domesticated plant and animal species for our food supply. Nevertheless, people continue to gather food which grows around their homes or they cultivate local varieties of food plants (as well as keep land races of domestic animals). Generally, wild varieties tend to be richer in micronutrients and bioactive secondary metabolites, which are produced in adaptation to local environmental conditions. These metabolites trigger further adaptive responses by producing 'protective', bioactive compounds which, when ingested, result in the transfer of protective effects to our organism.

The preservation of local knowledge for future generations as well as the identification of new nutraceuticals by means of characterizing plant extracts with potential health beneficial effects are the main objectives of this book. The first part therefore focuses on the ethnobotanical study of local food plants in selected regions of the Mediterranean. The biological-pharmacological effects of these plants on selected (mostly in vitro) targets of the central nervous system and the cardiovascular system make up the second part, highlighting the potential of these plants for developing novel health foods, herbal medicines or local products with beneficial effects on health.

Those interested in an integrated approach to the identification of new and health-beneficial foods will undoubtedly find this book a valuable source of information and an inspiration for new scientific approaches to this age-old topic.

KI 06650

Contents

www.karger.com/fonut

Forum of Nutrition, Vol. 59
Series Editor: Elmadfa, I. (Vienna)
ISSN 1660–0347

Local Mediterranean Food Plants and Nutraceuticals
Editors: Heinrich, M. (London); Müller, W.E. (Frankfurt); Galli, C. (Milano)
XII + 186 p., 24 fig., 23 tab., hard cover, 2006
CHF 228.– / EUR 163.– / USD 207.25
Prices subject to change
EUR price for Germany, USD price for USA only
ISBN-10: 3–8055–8124–6
ISBN-13: 978–3–8055–8124–0

KARGER

Order Form

Please send: ____ copy/ies

Postage and handling free with prepayment

Payment:
☐ Check enclosed ☐ Please bill me

Please charge to my credit card
☐ American Express ☐ Diners ☐ Eurocard
☐ MasterCard ☐ Visa

Card No.: ____________________

Exp. date: ____________________

Orders may be placed with any bookshop, subscription agency, directly with the publisher or through a Karger distributor.

Fax: +41 61 306 12 34

S. Karger AG, P.O. Box, CH–4009 Basel (Switzerland)
E-Mail orders@karger.ch, **www.karger.com**

Name/Address: ____________________

____

____

____

____

Date: ____________________

Signature: ____________________

Forschende Komplementärmedizin
Wissenschaft • Praxis • Perspektiven

Editorial

Forsch Komplementärmed 2007;17(suppl 1):VII–VIII

International Congress on Complementary Medicine Research

Munich, Germany, May 11–13, 2007

Dieter Melchart[1,2] George Lewith[3] Harald Walach[4] Wolfgang Weidenhammer[1] Klaus Linde[1]

[1] Centre for Complementary Medicine Research, Technical University Munich, Germany
[2] Division of Complementary Medicine, University Hospital Zurich, Switzerland
[3] Primary Care Group, CCS Division, University of Southampton, UK
[4] School of Social Sciences & Samueli Institute, University of Northampton, UK

The quantity and quality of research in complementary therapies has increased dramatically over the last decade in parallel with the expertise and intellectual capacity available for evaluating this challenging field. While CAM research is highly heterogeneous, many of the questions and problems within CAM are similar and researchers in general benefit enormously from exchanging ideas.

In 2000, the Centre for Complementary Medicine Research at the Technical University in Munich hosted a congress titled 'Evidence-Based Complementary Medicine – State of the Evidence and Methodological Challenges'. This event was organized in collaboration with the Centre for Alternative Medicine Research and Education, Beth Israel Deaconess Medical Centre, Harvard Medical School. A total of 80 abstracts from 14 different countries were submitted for presentation, of which 65 were accepted [1].

Now in 2007, the Centre for Complementary Medicine Research and the International Society for Complementary Medicine Research (ISCMR) have jointly-organized the International Congress on Complementary Medicine Research which will be held Munich in May. ISCMR was established in 2003 to foster co-operative and multidisciplinary research and development within complementary, traditional and integrative medicine. We hope that ISCMR will build on its success and continue to be a major international forum for researchers in the field. These continuing conferences will be the forum through which leading Complementary and Alternative Medicine (CAM) researchers can present their new research and discuss future strategies.

The conference organisers received a total of 264 abstracts from researchers in 26 different countries. In order to ensure scientific quality and to manage the Congress schedule, the Scientific Committee appointed a reviewing panel of 55 international expert volunteers. We are very grateful to them for their time, effort and expertise and would like to formally thank them for their work. Each abstract was evaluated by two external peer reviewers focussing on the criteria 'relevance', 'clarity of methods', 'quality of writing style' and 'global assessment'. All the abstracts were also read by two of the conference organizers; only if the external peer reviewers disagreed were the actual scores used to decide upon the submission's acceptance. Typical reasons for low scores were: prior publication of the submitted work, lack of clarity in the abstract, poor English, or a subject which might not be of interest to most Congress participants. We unfortunately had to reject 33% of the abstracts submitted, resulting in a scientific program of real excellence with 68 oral and 110 poster presentations.

The variety of research topics submitted has increased dramatically when compared to the 2000 conference (see table). While in 2000 'miscellaneous topics' comprised mainly methodological issues, these conferences' abstracts now contain a number of new discrete disciplines such as Anthroposophical Medicine and Mind-Body Medicine, as well as highlighting a number of is-

KARGER
Fax +49 761 4 52 07 14
E-mail Information@Karger.de
www.karger.com

Accessible online at:
www.karger.com/fok

sues within service delivery and medical integration. The relative predominance of acupuncture research seems to have diminished, although clinical trials on acupuncture have recently been of major importance in CAM research, particularly in Germany. This research has lead to a flood of recent well publicised international publications, so consequently there is little new work to present within this field. On the other hand, the increase in research topics within Traditional Chinese Medicine has been striking. It appears to us that both the quantity and quality of the submitted contributions has improved dramatically since 2000.

Topics	2000	2007
Classical Naturopathy	13%	10%
Acupuncture	22%	12%
Traditional Chinese Medicine	5%	13%
Phytotherapy	15%	16%
Homeopathy	9%	10%
Miscellaneous topics	36%	39%

The Congress programme will be centred around five distinguished keynote speeches. Hildebert Wagner from the University of Munich will present new research issues relating to the synergistic effects of phytomedicine. Heather Boon from the University of Toronto will discuss the relevance of qualitative methods in CAM research, utilising a study on the impact of the Canadian natural health product regulations as an example. The crucial subject of meaning or placebo effects will be discussed by Wayne Jonas, the director of the Samueli Institute. George Lewith from the University of Southampton will reflect on past lessons and future directions in acupuncture research. Dieter Melchart from the Technical University in Munich will give an overview on salutogenic mechanisms and their relevance for naturopathy and CAM in general.

Pre-conference workshops on whole systems research within herbal medicine, the methodology of systematic reviews and the networking of European CAM research groups will enrich this event.

The Centre for Complementary Medicine Research at the Technical University in Munich and the International Society for Complementary Medicine Research (ISCMR) are proud to host the International Congress on Complementary Medicine Research this year: next year the conference will be in Sydney Australia!

This supplementary issue of the FORSCHENDE KOMPLEMENTÄRMEDIZIN – RESEARCH IN COMPLEMENTARY MEDICINE covers all abstracts accepted and presented as talks or posters. The sequence of the abstracts follows the schedule of the Congress. The table of contents allows an easy navigation in order to identify individual contributions and each abstract is labelled by a code that corresponds to its designation in the Congress programme.

Special thanks go to the Erich Rothenfußer Foundation for their generous support of the Congress, and to the advertising companies for their support of this publication.

1 Forsch Komplementärmed 2000;7:29–58.

Forschende Komplementärmedizin
Wissenschaft • Praxis • Perspektiven

Abstracts

Forsch Komplementärmed 2007;14(suppl 1):1–53

PL1-1

Developing a research strategy for acupuncture

Lewith G
Primary Care Group, CCS Division, University of Southampton, UK

I will look at the evidence available to estimate both the specific and non-specific effect size of acupuncture and consider the placebo within acupuncture trials, as well as the value of both placebo controlled trials and pragmatic acupuncture studies. The recent contributions from the large German insurance studies of acupuncture in chronic pain have added very substantially to our understanding of this treatment modality. I will argue for an augmented, mixed methodology that integrates basic mechanism studies, including modern imaging techniques such as fMRI, quantitative and qualitative research as well as safety and health economic data to obtain a more rigorous understanding of the clinical practice of acupuncture. I hope that by taking a broad, patient-centred, whole systems and rigorous approach we may arrive at a realistic and thoughtful evaluation of its relative value in comparison to placebo treatment and conventional medicine, as well as its potential for integration into conventional health care. This lecture will be a thoughtful reflection on progress so far with suggested strategies for the future.

PL1-2

Newest issues in research of synergy effects and multidrug- and multitarget-therapy in phytomedicine

Wagner H
Center of Pharma Research, Department of Pharmacy, University of Munich, Germany

Many years of therapeutic experience with herbal drug combinations have shown that they possess better efficacy and reduced side-effects in comparison with single herbal drugs. The same is also true of standardized plant extracts as compared with single isolated constituents thereof. Detailed pharmological investigations using molecular biological assays have revealed that this better efficacy must be due to additive or potentiated synergy effects caused by the constituents of the extract combinations. Several examples show how these synergy effects can be determined. Further informations on mechanisms underlaying these synergy effects can be expected from investigations of the gene/protein expression profiles within the platform of genomic and proteomic technologies. Surprisingly, clinical studies have also shown that a series of herbal drug preparations were therapeutically equivalent to synthetic drugs and superior in terms of safety. The advantage of these drug combinations is that the single components of the mixture can be applied in doses of relatively low concentrations. The results of these investigations suggest that the new concept of multidrug therapy can be described as a multi-target therapy, in which each component affects a different molecular target, resulting in a multicausal treatment. This pharmacological and therapeutic superiority and advantage of herbal drug combinations serves at the same time as a legitimation for the application of standardized herbal drug combinations in general. The application of the „omic-technologies“ may lead to a change of paradigms towards the application of complex mixtures in medicine and open the new field of Phytogenomics-, and proteomics.

PL2-1

Placebo research: The evidence for healing practices

Jonas WB
Samueli Institute, Alexandria VA, USA

Placebo effects are often considered irrelevant at best and a nuisance at worst for determining what is valuable in medicine. In this talk, I argue that research that involves placebo provides critical information for how the mind, body, and culture heal. Following a newly proposed definition of placebo as a therapeutic meaning and context response, empirical evidence is reviewed which underlines the importance of these effects for developing a science of healing. It is likely that the effects due to the individual meaning and context of an intervention are an important factor of any treatment approach. It would be therapeutically desirable to maximize these factors and have good evidence on which to base healing interventions.

PL2-2

The neurobiology of complementary medicine: Reflex therapies and chronic pain

Musial F, Michalsen A, Dobos GJ
Chair of Complementary Medicine, University of Duisburg-Essen; Department of Internal and Integrative Medicine, Kliniken Essen-Mitte, Germany

There is increasing clinical evidence that reflex therapies such as massage, Gua Sha, cupping, wet packs etc. are helpful in reducing symptoms of chronic pain. However, the neurobiological basis of these effects has rarely been investigated even though the increasing knowledge of the pathophysiology of chronic pain syndromes allows for specific hypotheses. According to Jänig (2005) there are at least three mechanisms fostering the development of chronic and functional pain syndromes in the absence of a direct impairment of the nociceptive system: i) the environment of the nociceptor is altered (e.g. inflammation), while the nociceptor itself is intact; ii) neuroplastic changes in the spinal cord; iii) emotional and attentional states altering the processing of the pain signal. Furthermore, there is increasing evidence that negative emotions and stress alter pain perception through the affective-emotional pain pathway and that these mechanisms are also important for the understanding of visceral pain. Reflex therapies are likely able to influence chronic pain at the level of the nociceptor and the spinal cord. Moreover, it can be speculated that these therapies mimick the effect of "grooming" as a social intervention. Since it is well accepted that the positive effect of grooming has a neurobiological basis in non-human primates, its biosocial impact on well being and pain processing in humans may be underestimated. A synopsis of the neurobiological bases of pain perception, from the nociceptor up the spinal cord to brain mechanisms including the role of negative emotions and stress provides the basis for the investigation of the "way of action" of reflex therapies. Specific hypotheses on their neurobiological bases and methods suitable for their investigation are outlined. Further clarification of the mechanisms of action of reflex therapies will support their clinical evidence and add to our understanding of the neurobiology of complementary medicine.

KARGER
Fax +49 761 4 52 07 14
E-mail Information@Karger.de
www.karger.com

Accessible online at:
www.karger.com/fok

PL2-3

Ethical imperatives and obligation(s) for research in CAM: Can a core philosophical basis enable a truly integrative medicine?

Giordano J

Center for Clinical Bioethics, Georgetown University Medical Center and Samueli Institute, USA

Aims: This work addresses what philosophical and ethical bases, obligations and imperatives drive complementary and alternative medical research, and how satisfaction of these philosophical and moral conditions can enable a realistically integrative medicine. It argues that a core philosophy determines the ethical foundations of medicine, and compels and sustains the moral obligations for and in CAM research. **Methods:** The phenomenological method is used to describe the essence of medical practice, and show how the relational structure of the practice is critical to and supported by the moral obligations for progressive knowledge so as to satisfy both beneficence and non-maleficence along a continuum of normative and applied ethics. Through analysis of knowledge domains required for clinical practice, this work will posit the need for ongoing research in CAM, development and utilization of broader, yet no less rigorous research methodologies, and the importance of such studies to satisfy the epistemic, empirical, contextual and prudential dimensions upon which the ethics of the clinical encounter rely. **Results:** This work posits a deontic (rule-based) ethical framework that 1) constructs the general moral affirmations required of the practice of medicine, and 2) elucidates the importance of research-derived knowledge to the "structure and acts" of that practice. Yet, while necessary, rules for research and practice are not sufficient, and this deontic foundation also sustains the necessity of agent based ethics, and the importance of research, and research-derived knowledge to the therapeutic and moral agency of the clinician. **Conclusions:** Such research-based knowledge fulfills, and is consistent with the philosophical premises and moral obligations that best uphold the possibility for a truly "integrative" medicine as an individual and public good within pluralized societies. The development of heterodox approaches in research, education, practice, and need for supportive policy change(s) will be discussed to encourage considerations and dialogue for the future.

PL3-1

What outcome measures do we need? Development of the Canadian IN-CAM outcomes database

Verhoef M[1], Ware M[2], Dryden T[3], Weeks L[1], Gignac P[3], Mallory D[3], Ferguson L[2], Xu T[1], Brazier A[4]

[1]Department of Community Health Sciences, University of Calgary, Canada; [2]Departments of Anesthesia and Family Medicine, McGill University, Montreal, Canada; [3]Centre for Applied Research in Health, Technology & Education, School of Community and Health Studies, Centennial College, Toronto, Canada; [4]School of Nursing, University of British Columbia, Vancouver, Canada

Aims: Researchers evaluating the outcomes of CAM interventions must identify psychometrically sound, relevant outcome measures. Given the complexity of CAM interventions, in particular CAM whole systems, most such studies will need multiple outcome measures. Locating reliable, comprehensive information on a variety of outcome measures can be tedious and time consuming. Therefore, we identified the need for a web-based, comprehensive, searchable, practical and interactive CAM outcomes database. We will present the development and characteristics of such a database in Canada, as well as demonstrate its features and use. **Methods:** Based on a strategic CAM research planning meeting held by the Canadian Interdisciplinary Network for CAM Research (IN-CAM), a CAM outcomes workshop and a survey of CAM researchers, practitioners and educators, we developed a framework of relevant outcome domains and identified important features of a CAM outcomes database. **Results:** One hundred and sixty-four individuals responded to our email survey. Identified barriers to finding and using outcome measures included lack of existing measures that capture outcomes relevant to CAM, lack of a common resource, not knowing where to look and poor documentation in the literature. Following this survey, the research team held a consensus meeting to develop a framework of nine outcome domains based on the questionnaire responses. These include 1) physical, 2) psychological, 3) social and 4) spiritual aspects of the intervention, 5) holistic outcomes that encompass each of the physical, psychological, social and spiritual domains, 6) quality of life encompasses any two of the physical, psychological, social and spiritual domains, 7) individualized measures assess unique patient-centred outcomes for each research participant, 8) the process of healing and 9) the context of healing. **Discussion:** The IN-CAM Outcomes Database will assist CAM researchers in finding appropriate measures, and will encourage researchers to develop outcome measures in domains for which, thus far, no outcome instruments are available. While currently about 25 measures have been entered, database development is an ongoing process that most likely will continue for many years to come.

PL3-2

"At least we know it wasn't made in a bathtub": Exploring the impact of the Canadian natural health product regulations

Boon H

Faculty of Pharmacy, University of Toronto, Canada

All too often we implement policy changes without assessing their impact. After a brief introduction to Canada's new natural health product regulations, this presentation will focus on how the regulations are impacting a variety of key stakeholders including industry, complementary and alternative medicine practitioners, consumers, pharmacists and researchers. Data from each group were collected by an interdisciplinary team of researchers, graduate students, practitioners and policy-makers using qualitative interviews and focus groups. Key findings from each group will be reported. In addition, the strengths and weakness of using a qualitative approach will be discussed.

PL3-3

Salutogenesis and CAM

Melchart D

Centre for Complementary Medicine Research, Technical University Munich, Germany, and Division of Complementary Medicine, University Hospital Zurich, Switzerland

Many CAM-methods often offer salutogenic perspectives. Theories of salutogenesis are important as a basis for health promotion because the explanatory variables are formulated in terms of health resources. These resources are available to people (or are lacking) as physiological and personal resources, skills, sense of integrity etc at the individual level, or as living and environmental conditions in the external world. The theoretical models of salutogenesis have developed from stress theories, supplemented by disease management factors. Essentially, they are theories about the interplay of stresses and management strategies, risks and health resources. The author will introduce a comprehensive model for salutogenesis and CAM.

MA1-1

Integrated care in practice: Is acupuncture a useful adjunct to exercise-based physiotherapy for older adults with knee pain?

Foster NE[1], Thomas E[1], Barlas P[2], Hill J[1], Mason L[1], Young J[1], Hay EM[1]

[1]Primary Care Musculoskeletal Research Centre, Keele University, UK; [2]School of Health and Rehabilitation, Keele University, UK

Aims: In the UK, physiotherapists often use acupuncture for pain relief within packages of care for older adults with knee pain and osteoarthritis. We tested the effectiveness of adding acupuncture to a package of advice and exercise delivered by physiotherapists in primary care for these patients. **Methods:** This randomised controlled trial assigned adults aged 50 and over with knee pain to up to 6 advice and exercise sessions (A&E n=116); A&E plus true acupuncture (n=117) or A&E plus non-penetrating acupuncture (both delivered over 7 sessions) (n=119). In the acupuncture groups, 6 to 10 acupuncture points were selected from an agreed list. Primary outcome was change in the Western Ontario and McMaster Universities Osteoarthritis Index (WOMAC) pain sub-scale at 6 months. Secondary outcomes included WOMAC function, pain intensity and unpleasantness and treatment response. Follow-ups were at 2 and 6 weeks, 6 and 12 months. Analysis was by intention to treat. The researchers were blind to treatment allocation. Participants were told they would receive A&E and might receive one of two forms of acupuncture. **Results:** 352/1061 potentially eligible patients were recruited (mean age 63 yrs); 94% reached 6 month follow-up. Baseline WOMAC pain scores (mean (SD)) were 9.2 (3.8) and function scores were 30.7 (13.5). Mean reductions at 6 months were 2.28 (3.8) for A&E, 2.32 (3.6) for A&E plus true acupuncture and 2.53 (4.2) for A&E plus non-penetrating acupuncture. Compared with A&E alone, mean differences in WOMAC pain were -0·08 (95%CI: -1.0,0.9) for A&E plus true acupuncture and 0.25 (95%CI: -0.8,1.3) for A&E plus non-penetrating acupuncture. Similar differences were seen at other follow-ups. There were small, statistically significant reductions in pain intensity and unpleasantness for true acupuncture at 2 weeks and 6 weeks and for non-penetrating acupuncture at all follow-up points. The proportion of treatment responders at 6 months was 43% for A&E, 50% for A&E plus true acupuncture and 52% for A&E plus non-penetrating acupuncture. **Conclusions:** Acupuncture for older adults with knee pain delivered by physiotherapists provided no additional improvement in WOMAC pain scores compared with advice and exercise alone. Small benefits in pain intensity and unpleasantness were observed for both acupuncture groups, making it unlikely that this was due to acupuncture needling effects.

MA1-2

Acupuncture and physiotherapy for the treatment of painful shoulder: A multicentre randomised controlled trial

Vas J[1], Ortega C[2], Olmo MV[3], Mendez C[4], Perea-Milla E[5]

[1]Pain Treatment Unit, Centro de Salud Dos Hermanas, Distrito Sanitario Sevilla-Sur, Se villa, Spain; [2]Servicio de Rahabilitacion, Hospital Infanta Elena, Huelva, Spain; [3]Servicio de Rahabilitacion, Hospital Infanta Margarita, Cabra, Cordoba, Spain; [4]Direccion General de Calidad, Investigacón y Gestion del Conocimiento, Consejeria de Salud, Se villa, Spain; [5]Unidad de Apoyo a la Investigacion, Hospital Costa del Sol, Marbella, Malaga, Spain

Aim: To investigate the effectiveness of acupuncture in conjunction with physiotherapy for patients with painful shoulder. **Methods**: Randomised controlled multicentre study with blind evaluation by an independent observer and blind, independent analysis, carried out from January 2005 to December 2006, at five Rehabilitation Centres and a Pain Treatment Unit, in the context of primary healthcare in the Andalusian Public Health System (Spain), and a Rehabilitation Centre run by the Health Service of Murcia (Spain). The patients were randomly assigned to receive acupuncture in conjunction with physiotherapy or mock-TENS in conjunction with physiotherapy. Acupuncture and mock-TENS were administered by medical specialists and consisted of three sessions per patient over a period of three weeks. The physiotherapy was applied by trained physiotherapists and consisted of 15 sessions per patient over a period of three weeks. The primary result measure was taken to be the change observed on the Constant-Murley Scale (CMS) for functional assessment of the shoulder at 4 weeks and at 3, 6 and 12 months after the randomisation. **Results:** A total of 425 patients were included in the study; these were adults suffering unilateral subacromial syndrome (72.2% female), with a mean age (SD) of 55.7 (11.4) years; 325 of them had rotator cuff tendinitis, 52 had subacromial bursitis and 48 had, in addition, adhesive capsulitis (frozen shoulder). On completing the treatment, the mean score (SD) on the CMS had increased by 16.6 (15.6) points in the acupuncture group, compared with an increase of 10.6 (13.5) points in the control group; the mean difference between the two groups was statistically significant (-6.0 points; 95% CI -8.8 to -3.2 points; p<0.001). At three months after randomisation, the mean change from the baseline measure on the CMS was 25.4 (15.5) in the acupuncture group and 14.7 (18.0) in the control group, with a mean difference of -10.7 points (95% CI -14.1 to -7.3 points; p<0.001). On ending the treatment, 53% of the patients in the acupuncture group had reduced their consumption of analgesic medicaments, compared with 30% of those in the control group. **Conclusions:** Acupuncture in conjunction with physiotherapy improves shoulder functioning and reduces pain, to a greater extent than does physiotherapy alone. This improvement is accompanied by a corresponding reduction in the consumption of analgesic medicaments.

MA1-3

Clinical and economic effectiveness of acupuncture in patients with allergic asthma: A pragmatic randomised study

Brinkhaus B, Witt C, Reinhold T, Jena S, Willich SN

Institute for Social Medicine, Epidemiology, and Health Economics, Charité University Medical Center, Berlin, Germany

Background: The aim of the study was to evaluate the effectiveness and cost-effectiveness of acupuncture in addition to routine care in patients with allergic asthma compared to treatment with routine care alone. **Methods:** Adult patients with allergic asthma (disease duration > 6 months) were randomly allocated to a group receiving up to 15 acupuncture sessions over three months (ACU) or to a control group (CON) receiving no acupuncture. Study participants were allowed to receive additional usual medical care. By using standardised questionnaires we assessed asthma specific quality of life (AQLQ) and health related general quality of life (SF-36) at baseline and after three months. Data for direct costs and sick leave were provided by the health insurance fund. The cost-effectiveness-analysis was performed from an societal overall cost perspective. Incremental cost-effectiveness-ratios (ICER) were calculated based on the health related general quality adjusted life years (QALYs). **Results:** A total of 357 patients (184 acupuncture-group, 173 control-group; 42.6% men, age 48.2±13.9 years; 57.4% women, 45.0±12.5 years) were included in the study. At three months, the improvement of AQLQ was more pronounced in the ACU than in the CON (AQLQ: from 4.3±1.1 to 5.2±1.1; and from 4.5±0,9 to 4.6±1.2, p<0.001). ACU treatment was associated with higher overall costs compared to CON (p=0.002), mainly due to the acupuncture costs. There were more QALYs gained in the ACU compared to the CON (difference ACU - CON: 0.009±0.012). The incremental cost effectiveness ratio was 39,858 Euro/QALY gained. **Conclusions:** Treatment of patients with allergic asthma with acupuncture in addition to routine care was more effective than routine care alone and was cost effective in approximate 50% of all cases according to international cost-effectiveness threshold values of 50,000 Euro.

MA1-4

A comparison of endometrial vascularity in IVF patients after acupuncture treatment

So WS, Ehy NG, Wong YY

The University of Hong Kong

Aims: Despite recent advances in IVF treatment, the implantation potential of embryos remains low. Several studies showed a significant increase in IVF pregnancy rate following acupuncture but the underlying mechanism is largely unknown. The hypothesis is that there may be significant changes in endometrial vascularity after acupuncture. **Methods:** Vascularization index (VI), flow index (FI) and vascularization flow index (VFI) of endometrial and subendometrial regions were determined by three-dimensional ultrasound with power Doppler on the day of embryo transfer both before and after 25 minutes of acupuncture. **Results:** Although there were no significant changes in endometrial vascularity before and after acupuncture among 9 stimulated cycle patients and 7 natural cycle patients, a trend in the decline in subendometrial vascularity was shown, especially for the stimulated cycle patients. The mean changes in endometrial VI/FI/VFI were -16.5%, 17.8% and -12.5% respectively whereas the corresponding decreases in the 1mm and 5mm subendometrial regions were 13.2%, 17.2%, 8.3%; 17.8%, 7.4% and 16.6% respectively. **Conclusions:** Changing of endometrial and subendometrial blood flow may be one of the underlying mechanisms in increasing the IVF pregnancy rate after acupuncture.

MA1-5

Are experienced acupuncturists more successful?

Witt CM[1], Lüdtke R[2], Wegscheider K[3], Brinkhaus B[1], Willich SN[1]

[1]Institute for Social Medicine, Epidemiology and Health Economics, Charité University Medical Center; [2]Karl and Veronica Carstens Foundation, Germany; [3]Institute of Statistics and Econometrics, University of Hamburg, Germany

Aims: The aim was to quantify the influence of training and experience in the field of acupuncture on the outcome in patients with chronic pain. **Methods:** Patients visiting their physician because of chronic low back pain, headache, pain due to osteoarthritis of the knee or hip, or neck pain, who fulfilled predefined diagnosis-specific criteria, were included in four multi-centre randomized controlled studies. Patients in the acupuncture group received acupuncture immediately (on average 10 sessions), the patients in the control group did not receive acupuncture. All patients received routine care. We pooled the data and in order to identify factors affecting improvements we studied the 3-month change to baseline of the SF-36 bodily pain subscale, since this scale was identically determined for the different diagnoses. We fitted linear mixed models with physicians as random effect and several covariates on the physician and the patient level. We pre-specified the following characteristics of the physicians as potential confounders or effect modifiers: age, gender, years of professional experience, type of acupuncture diploma (140 vs. 350 hours), hours of acupuncture training, years of acupuncture experience, diagnosis in the context of traditional Chinese medicine, and percent of practice time with acupuncture treatment. **Results:** A total of 9990 patients (mean age 49.6±13.6 years, 68% female) were treated by 1760 physicians (mean age 46.8±7.1 years, 37% female). On average the physicians had 7.4±5.3 (range 1–33) years of acupuncture experience and their mean duration of acupuncture training was 280±239 hours (range 100–5000). The outcome was markedly improved when acupuncture was practiced. While several patient characteristics (bodily pain at baseline, diagnosis, age, education) were associated with bodily pain, none of the physician characteristics revealed a significant influence on the outcome, neither in the total population nor in the acupuncture group alone. **Conclusions:** In this analysis, physician characteristics such as training did not influence patients' outcome after acupuncture. Results might be interpreted as an indication that formal training has only a limited influence on treatment effect. So-called soft skills, which are difficult to measure, may probably play a more important role.

MA1-6

Acupuncture for post-stroke rehabilitation: A systematic review of randomized controlled clinical trials

Seely D[1,2], Wu P[1], Mills E[2]

[1]Department of Research and Clinical Epidemiology, The Canadian College of Naturopathic Medicine, Toronto, ON, Canada; [2]Institute of Medical Science, University of Toronto, Toronto, ON, Canada; [3]Centre for International Health and Human Rights Studies, Toronto, ON, Canada

Objective: In order to assess the efficacy of acupuncture in post-stroke rehabilitation, one must include all relevant trials. Thus far, systematic reviews on this topic have been affected by language bias. We aimed to reduce language bias by conducting a comprehensive analysis of all relevant trials with no limitation based on the language of publication. **Design:** Systematic review and meta-analysis of randomized controlled trials (RCTs) of acupuncture in post stroke rehabilitation. **Literature Search:** The following electronic databases were searched from inception to November 2006: MEDLINE, AMED, Alt HEALTH WATCH, CINAHL, Nursing and Allied Health Collection: Basic, Cochrane CENTRAL, and the Chinese database (CHKI). **Study selection:** Eligible studies included RCTs that evaluated the efficacy of acupuncture in adult patients with disability after stroke. **Data extraction:** We abstracted data on randomization, appropriateness of acupuncture rationale, methods of acupuncture including depth of insertion and needle type, patient characteristics, clinical status, frequency of treatment sessions, equality of co-interventions between groups, patient withdrawals, and the reliability of assessor and patient blinding. Outcome measurements included parameters of efficacy using various stroke evaluation criteria. Heterogeneity was assessed and a univariate meta-regression analysis was employed to determine if any of the above covariates predicted heterogeneity. **Results:** Twenty-one articles in Chinese and thirteen articles in English fit the inclusion criteria. Based on STRICTA criteria, the overall quality of the studies was relatively poor and sample sizes were small. The majority of studies reported a significant positive benefit of acupuncture in post stroke rehabilitation; five studies reported positive benefits in subgroup analyses and four studies reported no effectiveness. In Twenty trials, data was available for meta-analysis and meta-regression, the results of which yielded an odds ratio (OR) in favor of acupuncture compared to controls; OR = 5.57 (95%CI: 3.60-8.62; I2 = 43.4%). Based on the meta-regression; randomization, assessor blinding and the patient's clinical status may explain the outcome heterogeneity. **Conclusion:** RCTs demonstrate that acupuncture is an effective treatment for post-stroke rehabilitation. Our analysis provides further evidence on the utility of combining publications regardless of point of origin or language in meta-analysis. In addition to the outcome assessed, this study also demonstrates that randomization, assessor blinding, and the time at which the patient are treated could be important factors in evaluating the effectiveness of acupuncture for post-stroke rehabilitation.

MA2-1

Ginkgo biloba for mild to moderate dementia in the community: A pragmatic, randomised, parallel-group, double-blind, placebo-controlled trial

Fisher P[1], McCarney R[2], Iliffe S[3], van Haselen R[4], Griffin M[3], van der Meulen J[5], Warner J[2]

[1]Royal London Homoeopathic Hospital, London, UK; [2]Department of Psychological Medicine, Imperial College, London, UK; [3]Department of Primary Care and Population Sciences, UCL,UK; [4]International Institute for Integrated Medicine,France; [5]London School of Hygiene and Tropical Medicine, UK

Background: There is a need for safe, cheap and effective treatments for dementia which can be used in the early stages of the disease. Ginkgo biloba is a herbal medicine which has generated much interest; however its benefits remain unclear. **Methods:** We conducted a community-based, pragmatic, randomised, double-blind, parallel-group trial in which participants with mild-to-moderate dementia (Mini Mental State Examination [MMSE] score 12-26) received a standardised extract of Ginkgo biloba (EGb 761®,120mg daily) or a placebo control for six months. Our primary outcomes were cognitive functioning (ADAS-Cog) and participant and carer-rated quality of life (QOL-AD). The main analysis was Intention to Treat using multiple imputation techniques for the missing data. **Results:** We recruited 176 participants, mainly through general practices. In the ANCOVA model with baseline score as a co-variate (n=176), Ginkgo did not have a significant effect on outcome at six months on either the ADAS-Cog score (p=0.392), the participant-rated QOL-AD score (p=0.787) nor the carer-rated QOL-AD score (p=0.222). Analyses with evaluable data and per protocol showed similar results. A total of 63 adverse events were recorded (29 in the placebo group, 28 in the Ginkgo group). **Conclusion:** We found no evidence that a standard dose of high purity Ginkgo biloba confers benefit in mild-moderate dementia over six months. The recruitment shortfall means a type II error is a possibility, although no trends were detected in the data. Based on our findings, Ginkgo is unlikely to confer benefit of any clinical significance and the implication of this is that we do not recommend its use in routine dementia care.

MA2-2

Choosing between NSAID and Arnica for topical treatment of osteoarthritis in hands: Does it matter?

Widrig R[1], Suter A[2], Saller R[3], Melzer J[3]

[1]Rheumatology clinic, St Gallen, Switzerland; [2]Bioforce AG, Roggwil, Switzerland; [3]Institute of Complementary Medicine, Department of Internal Medicine, University Hospital Zurich, Switzerland

Background: The use of topical non-steroidal anti-inflammatory preparations for symptom relief in osteoarthritis has spiralled recently to a point at which gel, cream and spray are commonly used. **Objective:** To evaluate the effects of ibuprofen (5%) and arnica (50 g tincture / 100 g, DER 1:20) as gel preparations in patients with radiologically confirmed and symptomatically active osteoarthritis of interphalangeal joints of hands. **Methods:** Randomised, controlled, double-blind study in 204 patients in 20 clinics, to ascertain differences in pain relief and hand function. Diagnosis was according to established criteria; primary endpoints were pain intensity measured by visual analogue scale (VAS) and hand function by validated Hand Algofunctional Index (HAI); statistical design for non-inferiority as per regulatory guideline for statistical testing of topical preparations. **Results:** Although both treatments showed improvements in all parameters, the results did not show a therapeutic advantage of ibuprofen over arnica. Pain improvement was 23.9±23.3 and 26.6±22.4 mm (VAS) in the ibuprofen and arnica group (Δ=3.4; [95.2% CI: -2.9; 9.7]) and improvement in functional capacity was 4.6±3.1 and 4.3±3.6 points (HAI) (Δ=-0.2; [CI 95.2%: -1.3; 0.8]), respectively. None of the secondary end points (e.g. number of painful joints, morning stiffness intensity and duration; analgesic consumption) differed between treatments. Adverse events were reported by 6 patients (6.1%) on ibuprofen and by 5 patients (4.8%) on arnica. **Conclusions:** Our results confirm that this herbal preparation of arnica is not inferior to ibuprofen when used topically to treat osteoarthritis of hands. Both treatments can ameliorate symptoms and are well tolerated.

MA2-3

Complex estimation of biological activity for individual herbal substances and their combinations

Lagunin AA, Gomazkov OA, Dergacheva LI, Shevchenko TV, Filimonov DA, Poroikov VV

Institute of Biomedical Chemistry of Rus. Acad. Med. Sci., Moscow, Russia

Aims: Development and validation of computer-aided methods for complex estimation of probable pharmacological effects and biochemical mechanisms of action for individual herbal substances and their combinations. **Methods:** We developed computer program PASS (Prediction of Activity Spectra for Substances, http://www.ibmc.msk.ru/PASS). On the basis of structural formula of chemical compound PASS predicts more than 2500 pharmacological effects, mechanisms of actions, specific toxicity, metabolic terms with average accuracy about 92%. PASS predictions for individual herbal substances can be analyzed with computer program PharmaExpert, which provides the means for estimation of activity-activity relationships. Using PharmaExpert one can identify probable interactions between the individual substances; thus obtaining general biological activity profiles for their combinations/mixtures. **Results:** Biological activity spectra were predicted for different phytoflavonoides (quercetine, resveratrol, etc.) as well as for other substances from the appropriate medicinal plants. On the basis of this data it was demonstrated a wide pharmacotherapeutical application of individual herbal substances and their combinations. Adverse/toxic effects predicted for some individual substances can be diminished by the opposite actions of other components in herbal extracts. It is also shown that some adverse/toxic effects of chemotherapeutical drugs can be compensated by application of herbal medicines. **Conclusions:** Computer-aided methods of biological activity estimation for individual herbal substances and their combinations provide the strong basis for their use in Complementary Medicine.

MA2-4

Herb-drug interactions: Warfarin anti-coagulant randomised clinical trials

Roufogalis BD[1], Mohammed Abdul MI[1], Jiang X[1], Liauw WS[2], Williams KM[2], Day RO[2], McLachlan AJ[1,3]

[1]Faculty of Pharmacy, University of Sydney, Sydney, NSW, Australia; [2]Clinical Trials Centre, St Vincent's Hospital, Darlinghurst and University of NSW, NSW, Australia; [3]Centre for Education and Research on Ageing, Concord Hospital, NSW, Australia

Background: Herbal medicines have potential to interact with warfarin, which could have a fatal outcome **Aim:** This study aimed to investigate pharmacokinetic and pharmacodynamic interactions between the anti-coagulant warfarin and four commonly used herbal medicines; cranberry, garlic, echinacea and policosanol. **Methods:** Two randomised, three treatment, cross over, clinical trials (trial 1- cranberry and garlic; trial 2- echinacea and policosanol) were performed involving 12 healthy, non smoking male subjects in each trial. Each subject in randomised order received and was crossed over to: 25 mg warfarin alone, 25 mg of warfarin after 2 weeks of multiple doses of the first herb and 25 mg of warfarin after 2 weeks of multiple doses of the other herb in each trial. Herbs were continued for another 1 week after warfarin administration in the herbal treatment periods and blood samples were collected for up to 168 h of warfarin administration. Pharmacodynamics (INR) and pharmacokinetics (AUC) of warfarin were compared between warfarin only treatment and warfarin and herbal treatment periods and reported as mean ratio and 90% confidence interval (CI) ratio. Values within 0.8 to 1.25 were considered not to show a significant change. **Results**: Cranberry significantly increased INR of warfarin when given along with warfarin, with mean ratio and 90% CI ratio of 1.28 (1.06–1.54). None of the other herbs altered INR when given along with warfarin, with mean ratio and 90% CI of 0.99 (0.82–1.19) for garlic; 1.09 (0.90–1.31) for policosanol; 1.01 (0.84–1.22) for echinacea. Neither cranberry nor garlic altered AUC of S-warfarin, with mean ratio and 90% CI of 1.05 (1.00–1.02); 1.08 (0.98–1.18), respectively. Neither echinacea nor policosanol altered AUC of S-warfarin (N=5). **Conclusions:** Cranberry increased the warfarin pharmacodynamic response by an unknown mechanism. However other herbs studied had less propensity to interact with warfarin. Similar studies in patients are needed to elucidate the clinical significance of these herb warfarin combinations.

MA2-5

Changing with herbs: Treatment of menopausal symptoms by qualified herbal practitioners

Green J[1], Denham A[2], Ingram J[3], Hawkey S[4], Greenwood R[3]

[1]National Institute of Medical Herbalists, Exeter, UK; [2]Department of Nursing, University of Central Lancashire, Preston, UK; [3]Bristol Research & Development Support Unit, Bristol Royal Infirmary, UK; [4]School of Health and Bioscience, University of East London, London, UK

Aims: To assess the effectiveness of treatment of menopausal symptoms by qualified herbal practitioners. **Methods:** A sample of 45 women from one UK urban GP practice was recruited into a pilot prospective randomised, waiting-list controlled trial. Participants were aged 46-59, experiencing self-defined menopausal symptoms and no menstrual bleeding for 3 months. Exclusion criteria were: use of hormone replacement therapy, oral contraception, "natural progesterone cream", tamoxifen, current complementary treatment for the menopause, or general anaesthesia within three months. Women who had received medical advice to take HRT due to risk of osteoporosis, and those who had received psychiatric treatment within 3 months were also excluded. The 45 participants were block randomised into a treatment group (n=15) who received a course of individualised treatment from one of 3 herbal practitioners, and control group (n=30) who were offered treatment after waiting 4 months. Treatment involved a series of 6 consultations over 5 months including discussion of diet, lifestyle, and individualised herbal prescription, adjusted if required at each consultation. Change in menopausal symptoms was measured in both groups using the validated Greene Climacteric Scale. Scores are grouped as vasomotor (hot flushes, night sweats), psychological (anxiety, depression), somatic, libido, and total of all symptoms. Analysis of variance was used to compare both groups across time. Measure Yourself Medical Outcomes Profile was also used to record changes in self-defined most troublesome symptoms. **Results:** 44 participants completed the trial. The treatment group demonstrated a statistically significant reduction in menopausal symptoms compared to the control group. Total scores for menopausal symptoms were reduced (p=0.001), as were vasomotor scores (p=0.001) and libido increased (p=0.005) in the group receiving herbal treatment. **Conclusion:** The treatment package from herbal practitioners improved menopausal symptoms, particularly hot flushes and low libido. This offers evidence to support treatment choices other than hormone replacement therapy (HRT). (Trial registration ISRCTN42406364)

MA2-6

Findings from a placebo controlled trial of hypericum perforatum for attention deficit hyperactivity disorder in children and adolescents

Weber W[1], VanderStoep A[2,3], McCarty R[1], Weiss NS[2], Biederman J[4,5], McClellan J[3]

[1]School of Naturopathic Medicine, Bastyr University, Kenmore, USA; [2]Department of Epidemiology, University of Washington, Seattle, USA; [3]Department of Psychiatry and Behavioral Sciences, University of Washington, Seattle, USA; [4]Department of Pediatric Psychopharmacology, Massachusetts General Hospital, Boston, USA; [5]Department of Psychiatry, Harvard University, Boston, USA

Aims: In the United States, it is estimated that Attention Deficit Hyperactivity Disorder (ADHD) affects 3-10% of children and adolescents. Many parents seek out complementary or alternative therapies for their children with ADHD. St. John s Wort is one of the top three botanicals used for children with this condition. **Methods:** A placebo controlled trial was conducted to determine the safety and efficacy of Hypericum perforatum (St. John's Wort) for the treatment of ADHD in children aged 6-17 years. The ADHD-IV Rating Scale (RS) was used as the primary measure for ADHD symptoms and was completed at all study visits. The Clinical Global Impression (CGI) and Severity scales were completed at weeks 4 and 8. In addition, potential adverse reactions including rash, nausea/vomiting, headache, and sunburn were recorded at each study visit. Other medications for ADHD were not allowed during the trial. **Results:** A total of 54 participants were randomized to study medication, with 27 in each group. Mean age of participants was 9.9 years, and the mean duration of ADHD symptoms for participants was 6.5 years. Only 40% of participants had previously been treated with pharmaceutical medications for ADHD symptoms. No significant difference was found in the change in ADHD-IV RS measures of inattention or hyperactivity between the Hypericum and placebo groups (inattention improved 2.6 points Hypericum vs. 3.2 pts placebo, p=0.68; hyperactivity improved 1.8 pts Hypericum vs. 2.0 pts placebo, p=0.89). No difference was found in the proportion of participants with greater than 25% improvement in any of the ADHD-IV RS measures or improvement (score of 2 or less) on the CGI scale (Hypericum 44.4% and placebo 51.9%, p=0.59). Among participants who completed the clinical trial according to protocol (81.5% in Hypericum vs. 70.4% in placebo groups, p=0.32), there were no differences in the improvements on either scale between the groups. No difference between groups was found in the total number of participants who experienced a potential adverse effect during the study period (Hypericum 25.9% and placebo 37.0%, p=0.38), nor was there an appreciable difference in the incidence of individual adverse events between groups. **Conclusions:** The results of this trial do not support the use of Hypericum to treat the symptoms of ADHD in children.

MA3-1

Anthroposophic mistletoe therapy in cancer: A systematic review of prospective clinical trials

Kienle GS, Kiene H

Institute for Applied Epistemology and Medical Methodology, Freiburg/Bad Krozingen, Germany

Background: Anthroposophic mistletoe therapy is a widely used complementary cancer treatment. **Objective:** To evaluate prospective clinical trials on the effectiveness of anthroposophic mistletoe therapy for cancer. **Design:** Systematic review. **Material and Methods:** Search of 9 electronic databases, reference lists and extensive expert consultations. Criteria-based assessment of methodological study quality. **Results:** 16 randomized (RCT) and 9 non-randomized (N-RCT) controlled trials were identified that investigated mistletoe treatment of malignant diseases. Statistically significant benefit for survival was reported in 8 of 17 trials (in 5 of 10 RCTs), for disease-free survival and tumour recurrence in none of 2 RCTs, for remission of tumour and malignant effusion in 1 RCT and 1 N-RCT of 4 controlled trials, for quality of life (QoL) in 3 of 5 RCTs, and for QoL and reduction of side effects of cytoreductive therapies (chemotherapy, radiation or surgery) in 5 of 7 trials (3 of 5 RCTs). Methodological quality of the controlled trials differed substantially; some had major limitations while others were reasonably well conducted. 12 single-arm cohort studies were identified. 5 of 7 studies found substantial tumour remission in various cancers, one study reported remission of CIN, and 4 studies remission of malignant pleural effusion or ascites. Quality of reporting in these cohort studies was mostly reasonably good. Mistletoe application was well tolerated. **Conclusions:** Regarding quality of studies and consistency of results, the best evidence for efficacy of mistletoe therapy exists for improvement of QoL and reduction of side effects of cytotoxic therapies (chemotherapy, radiation). Survival benefit has been shown but not beyond critique. Tumour remissions are described in cohort studies that investigate the application of high dose or local mistletoe extracts. As several reasonably well-conducted studies indicate beneficial effects, further properly designed trials should be encouraged to investigate clinical efficacy and its possible dependency on the mode of application.

MA3-2

Prospective controlled cohort studies in matched-pair design on long-term therapy of cervical, corpus uteri and ovarian cancer patients with a mistletoe preparation (Iscador)

Grossarth-Maticek R[1], Ziegler R[2]

[1]Institute for Preventive Medicine, European Center for Peace and Development (ECPD), Heidelberg, Germany;
[2]Society for Cancer Research, Institute Hiscia, Arlesheim, Switzerland

Aims: Mistletoe preparations such as Iscador are in common use as complementary medications, particularly for solid cancers. Does the long-term application of a complementary therapy with the mistletoe preparation Iscador show any effect in prospective studies on survival or psychosomatic self-regulation of patients with cervical, corpus uteri or ovarian cancer? **Methods:** Prospective recruitment and long-term follow-up in the following controlled 11 cohort studies. A) 5 Randomised matched-pair studies: Patients without/with distant metastases from cervical (0 pairs/19 pairs), corpus uteri (30 pairs/26 pairs) or ovarian cancer (21 pairs/20 pairs) that never used any kind of mistletoe therapy were matched for prognostic factors. By paired random allocation, one patient of a pair received a suggestion of mistletoe therapy to be applied by the attending physician. B) 6 non-randomised matched-pair studies: Cervical (102 pairs/66 pairs), corpus uteri (103 pairs/95 pairs) and ovarian (75 pairs/62 pairs) cancer patients without/with metastases that already received mistletoe (Iscador) therapy were matched by the same criteria to control patients without Iscador therapy. **Results:** 1. Overall survival: 2 from 5 randomised studies showed a significant effect (hazard ratio estimate and 95% confidence interval): Corpus uteri cancer without metastases 0.36 (0.16, 0.82), ovarian cancer with metastases 0.33 (0.12, 0.92). In 5 from 6 non-randomised studies, the results (adjusted for relevant prognostic variables) were significant. 2. Within 12 months self-regulation rises significantly in the Iscador group compared to the control group in all 6 studies that measured this effect: Randomised studies with cervical, corpus uteri or ovarian cancer without metastases: estimate of the median difference and 95% confidence interval: 0.70 (0.15, 1.05), 0.40 (0.15, 0.70) and 0.58 (0.30, 0.90). Non-randomised studies with cervical, corpus uteri or ovarian cancer without metastases: 0.25 (0.15, 0.35), 0.70 (0.25, 1.15) and 0.30 (0.05, 0.65). **Conclusions:** The mistletoe preparation Iscador might have a prolonging effect on overall survival of cervical, corpus uteri and ovarian cancer patients of all stages. In the short term, self-regulation rises significantly more under complementary Iscador therapy than under conventional therapy alone in all studies measured.

MA3-3

Dynamisation of mistletoe (Viscum album L.) by means of an Anthroposophical pharmaceutical process

Baumgartner S[1, 2], Flückiger H[1], Heertsch A[1], Jäggy C[1], Schaller G[1], Scherr C[1], Urech K[1]

[1]Society for Cancer Research, Institute Hiscia, Arlesheim, Switzerland;
[2]Institute of Complementary Medicine KIKOM, University of Berne, Switzerland

Aims: Aqueous extracts of European mistletoe (Viscum album L.) such as Iscador® are widely used in CAM cancer care. Rudolf Steiner, the founder of Anthroposophical Medicine, introduced mistletoe as specific cancer remedy into medicine. He suggested using injectable extracts of mistletoe, prepared from summer and winter harvests and subsequent extraction. Both extracts are to be mixed together by a special dynamisation procedure with the aim of increasing the anti-cancer efficacy. This pharmaceutical process is based upon a mixture of the extracts in the edge of a disk rotating with 10,000 rpm. We set out to identify the effects of this specific process, designed and realised by staff members of the "Society for Cancer Research" in Arlesheim, Switzerland. **Methods:** We investigated this mistletoe dynamisation process by comparing preclinical effects of three preparations: i) water (zero control), ii) viscum (viscum control, summer and winter extracts stirred together manually), and iii) dynamised viscum (summer and winter extracts mixed on the rotating disk). Different preclinical approaches were used: analytical composition, toxicity in cancer cell lines, and botanical whole system bioassays with and without noxae. **Results:** The investigated dynamisation process of mistletoe (1) does not change the concentration of pharmacological compounds such as lectins and viscotoxins, (2) does not change the antiproliferative effects of the extract in cancer cell lines (Molt4, Yoshida), (3) has small effects when applied on healthy plants, (4) approximately doubles the protective effect against external noxae (UV-radiation, colchicine, Agrobacterium tumefaciens) that lead to phenomenological malformations in plants, and (5) has no detectable effect in plant systems with external noxae leading to general damage without apparent malformations (arsenic, Pseudomonas syringae). **Conclusions:** Whole system bioassays such as plants, but not cancer cell lines, seem to be suited to show effects of the described dynamisation process of mistletoe. The procedure seems to result in extracts, which protect the plants from stressors leading to morphological malformations and strengthen the plant organisms as a whole.

MA3-4

The potential of a mistletoe extract to alleviate adverse effects of cancer chemotherapy: An in-vitro study

Burkhart J[1,2], Wälchli C[2,3], Heusser P[2], Andres AC[1], Baumgartner S[2,3]

[1]Department of Clinical Research, Faculty of Medicine, University of Berne, Switzerland; [2]Institute of Complementary Medicine KIKOM, University of Berne, Switzerland; [3]Society for Cancer Research, Institute Hiscia, Arlesheim, Switzerland

Aims: Mistletoe extracts have been shown to provide DNA stabilising effects in human peripheral blood mononuclear cells (PBMC) in vitro. We investigated the effect of a mistletoe extract (Iscador P) on unstimulated PBMC of healthy blood donors with and without concomitant treatment with cyclophosphamide. Furthermore we compared the behaviour of normal PBMC with that of cancerous lymphocytes. **Methods:** The experiments were carried out with PBMC of healthy blood donors and the T-leukemia cell line Jurkat. The cells were pre-incubated with mistletoe extract for 60–65 hours. 4-Hydroperoxycylophosphamide (4-HPC), the active metabolite of cyclophosphamide, was subsequently added and the cells incubated with 4-HPC for 2 hours. Cell viability and cell replication were measured with spectrophotometric tests (WST-1 reduction and BrdU incorporation, respectively). All experiments were blinded and randomised. **Results:** PBMC: Mistletoe extract (100 µg/ml) alone had a stimulating effect on cell viability and cell replication of +125% and +24%, respectively, referred to the mistletoe untreated cells (100%, $p<0.001$). Mistletoe extract in combination with 4-HPC had a stimulating effect of +125% on cell viability and of +152% on cell replication referred to the mistletoe untreated cells (100%, $p<0.001$). Thus, the mistletoe extract effect on cell replication was enhanced in 4-HPC treated cells (protective effect). Jurkat: No stimulating effect of the mistletoe extract could be shown in Jurkat cells with the assays used, neither with mistletoe extract alone nor in combination with 4-HPC. On the contrary, the mistletoe extract seemed to reinforce the cytotoxic effect of 4-HPC in Jurkat cells treated with mistletoe extract and 4-HPC (-4% on cell viability, $p<0.01$, and -15% on cell replication, $p<0.001$). **Conclusions:** Mistletoe extract (Iscador P) exerts in vitro a strong stimulating effect on healthy PBMC but not on malignant cells. When applied in combination with 4-HPC, it seems to protect healthy PBMC from the cytostatic effect of 4-HPC regarding replication. Again, this effect is restricted to healthy, non-cancerous cells. It needs to be investigated if the observed effects are due to a DNA stabilising effect, an improvement of the DNA repair, or another mechanism. The results motivate further clinical investigation of mistletoe extract (Iscador P) as an adjuvant in cancer therapy.

MA3-5

Relief of symptoms in female patients with a hypotensive symptom complex treated with Cardiodoron® – results of a randomized double-blind controlled study

Mayrhoffer M, Frühwirth M, Avian A, Grote V, Köhldorfer P, Kelz C, Meisermann T, Schwarz R, Salameh B, Winker R, Petzl D, Schwarz K, Schöber M, Ramos M, Moser M

Practicing doctor in Klagenfurt, Austria, in cooperation with Joanneum Research Institute of Non-Invasive Diagnosis

Aims: To test the efficacy and safety of Cardiodoron® (consisting of extracts from Primula officinalis, Onopordon acanthium, and Hyoscyamus niger) in the treatment of a hypotensive symptom complex in female patients. **Methods:** Sixty women (14–45 years) with hypotensive autonomic dysregulation symptoms including immediate or late orthostatic intolerance, blurred vision, physical weakness, fatigue, or cold limbs took part in this joint study of Joanneum Research and the Medical Universities of Vienna and Graz, Austria. They were recruited at three doctors practices and the clinical Department of Occupational Medicine Vienna. Patients were treated double blind with either Cardiodoron® or a Placebo orally in a dose of 20 drops 3 times a day for 8 weeks. General medical advice, e.g. regarding fluid and salt intake, was allowed in both groups. A questionnaire of symptoms (von Zerssen's symptom list) was filled out weekly throughout the study. Heart rate variability (HRV) was assessed by six 24h-Holter-ECG recordings, sleep quality by questionnaires: 2 times before treatment, during the third and sixth week of treatment, and 1 and 4 weeks after treatment. **Results:** Data of 57 patients were analyzed. The symptom score before treatment showed a value of 23.2 (Cardiodoron group) vs 22.5 (Placebo group) compared to the reference value of 15.5 in a german population of healthy females, and improved in both groups. The improvement was significantly higher in the Cardiodoron group (47%, to a score of 12.2 post medication) than in the control group (24%, to 17.0 post placebo). Besides the reduction of typical symptoms, back pain and sleep related problems improved. Despite of randomization, HRV was better in the Cardiodoron group right from the beginning, yet there were small additional improvements in nightly HRV parameters during the treatment phase. **Conclusions:** Cardiodoron® was more effective in treating the hypotensive symptom complex than placebo, and the effects remained at least four weeks after treatment. We do not suppose an unidirectional but a normalizing effect on autonomic regulation which will be further explored based on the collected data.

MA3-6

EVAMED – a prescription-based electronic pharmacovigilance system in complementary medicine

Jeschke E[1], Buchwald D[1], Lüke C[1], Tabali M[1], Ostermann T[2], Matthes H[1]

[1]Research Institute and Community Hospital Havelhoehe, Germany; [2]Department of Medical Theory and Complementary Medicine, University of Witten/Herdecke, Germany

Aims: Although there is evidence that herbal medicines can cause serious adverse reactions (ADRs), there is still a lack of knowledge about ADRs of Complementary and Alternative Medicines (CAM) in general practise. Hence, there is a need for a qualified reporting system for adverse events of CAM based on the number of patients treated with a given medicine. Therefore, we developed an electronic system for the continuous report of all prescriptions as well as ADRs if they occurred. **Material and Methods:** Based on a web oriented database system, EvaMed can easily be connected to the data of usual practice-software of physicians. Both, documentation and classification of ADRs are based on the WHO-standards of adverse reaction terminology (WHO-ART) and the grade of severity (from 1=light to 4=severe). **Results:** Since September 2004, data of 35 German anthroposophically oriented physicians have been collected. So far, a total of 294,037 prescriptions (for 62,685 patients, 60% female, children: 51%) were documented. They comprised 542,983 prescribed medicines (42% allopathic, 43% anthroposophical, 8% homeopathic, 7% herbal). Until September 2006 ADRs were reported in 288 cases (WHO-grade I: 41.3%, II: 46.5%, III: 10.8% and IV: 1.4%). In total, 74 cases were associated with anthroposophical therapies (25.7%). 12 (4.2%) of all ADRs where classified to serious but none of them was related to CAM-therapies. **Conclusion:** The described system for the collection and documentation of ADRs has proved effective for the evaluation of reported ADRs in close cooperation between prescribing physicians and the study center. General standards for the collection, transfer and evaluation of data can be used in any other environment. They also may contribute to an effective Pharmacovigilance system within the European Union. Acknowledgements: The EvaMed project is sponsored with a grant of the SAG-Foundation and financially supported by WALA and WELEDA.

MA4-1

Randomised, controlled, multicenter pilot study comparing qigong and back school for elderly patients with chronic neck pain

Wiedemann AM[1], von Trott P[1], Lüdtke R[2], Willich SN[1], Witt CM[1]

[1]Institute for Social Medicine, Epidemiology and Health Economics, Charité University Medical Center; [2]Karl and Veronica Carstens Foundation, Germany

Aims. In a randomised controlled trial we evaluated whether qigong is more effective compared to no treatment or to back school in elderly patients with chronic neck pain. **Methods:** Patients (age ≥ 55) with chronic neck pain (duration >6 months) and average pain at baseline of at least 20 mm on a 100 mm Visual Analogue Scale (VAS) were randomised to qigong, back school (each 24 sessions of 45min over a period of 3 months) or a waiting list group (no treatment). Patients completed standardised questionnaires at baseline and after 3 and 6 months. Main outcome measure was neck pain measured on the VAS (0–100 mm) after 3 months. Secondary outcome parameters were 'neck pain and disability' (Neck pain and Disability Scale by Wheeler; NPAD) and quality of life (SF-36). For statistical analysis we used multivariate repeated measurement ANCOVA (adjusted for baseline and patient expectation). Missing data were replaced using multiple imputations. **Results:** A total of 117 patients (95% female, mean age 76±8 years) were included in the intention-to-treat analysis. The average duration of neck pain was 20 years. After 3 months for neck pain no significant differences were observed between qigong and waiting list (mean estimated difference on the VAS -11 mm (confidence interval -24.0; 2.1), p=0.099) and between qigong and back school (-2.5 mm (-15.4; 10.3), p=0.699). Results for 'neck pain and disability' were similar (qigong vs. waiting list mean estimated difference on the NPAD -6.7 (-15.4; 2.1), p=0.135; qigong vs. back school difference 2.3 (-6.2; 10.8); p=0.600)). In addition for quality of life no significant differences between groups were observed. **Conclusion:** In this pilot study including elderly patients with long term chronic neck pain practicing qigong for 3 months had no relevant impact on neck pain, disability and quality of life if compared with no treatment. Further studies should enlarge the treatment period and the sample size and include patients with shorter disease duration.

MA4-2

The effect of external Qigong therapy on post-cardiovascular surgery pain, wound healing, and length of hospital stay

Warber SL, Gillespie BW, Ai A, Peterson C, Bolling SF

University of Michigan Integrative Medicine, Ann Arbor, USA

Aims: In cardiovascular surgery, pain control and wound healing are important patient-centered outcomes, and hospital length of stay is an important economic consideration. Previous studies of biofield energy therapy have shown promise in both pain control and improved wound healing. Our purpose was to examine the effect of external Qigong, a traditional Chinese energy therapy, on pain, wound healing, and length of hospital stay following cardiovascular surgery. **Methods:** We carried out a randomized clinical trial of Qigong therapy, mimic Qigong therapy, and standard medical care in 427 patients undergoing cardiovascular surgery at the University of Michigan Medical Center. Twenty-seven patients dropped out before surgery, never had surgery, or died in the peri-operative period. Qigong and mimic therapy were administered in 4 daily 1-hour sessions beginning immediately post surgery. Outcomes collected over the 4 days after surgery included self-reported modified Brief Pain Inventory, pain medication used, and ordinal wound-healing scales for the thorax or sternum. Length of hospital stay was measured from the day of surgery until discharge. Statistical analyses included chi-squared tests and repeated measures logistic and linear regressions. **Results:** For worst post-surgical pain, there was a significant difference between groups across days 2-4 (p=0.046) with the mimic group experiencing less pain. No significant differences were found between groups for average pain, chest pain, leg pain, or use of pain medications. For thoracic wounds, the frequency of non-zero wound scores by post-op day showed no significant differences between treatment groups (p=0.37). When length of stay was categorized into intervals of ≤4, 5–7, 8–14, and ≥15 days, no significant differences between treatment groups were observed (p=0.55). There were no differences between groups on frequency of adverse events or deaths. **Conclusions:** These results show that external Qigong is not effective for post-operative cardiac patients. Any future work in this area should focus on mechanistic and measurement issues.

MA4-3

Development and validation of an oriental medicine diagnostic instrument

Conboy LA[1,2], Schnyer RN[1,2], Legedza A[3], McKnight P[4], Kerr C[1,2], Kaptchuk TJ[1], Wayne P M[1,2]

[1]Osher Institute, Harvard Medical School, Boston, USA; [2]New England School of Acupuncture, Watertown, USA; [3]Beth Israel Deaconess Medical Center, Boston, USA; [4]George Mason University, Fairfax, USA

This project built on previous work operationalizing the Oriental Medicine (OM) diagnostic process to produce a tool for use in clinical trials of acupuncture to characterize the study population within the framework of OM. Using a Delphi process we refined a previously developed intake instrument that has been used in several clinical trials of acupuncture, in order to produce an OM diagnostic tool called the TEAMSI-TCM (Traditional East Asian Medicine Structure Interview). We tested the reliability and validity of this instrument, in order to increase the acceptance of the integration of OM into biomedical clinical research. The use of the TEAMSI-TCM in the selection of protocols and in the discussion and analysis of the results of an OM trial will provide essential information about the observed effects of the intervention and is an essential step in informing future practice and research. TEAMSI-TCM will make possible the systematic collection of these data and will facilitate the critical evaluation of the OM research literature. This presentation focuses on the validity data collected through interviews and surveys of the 40 practitioners who participated in the process. Two independent coders analyzed the transcripts and survey data and found that the new tool strongly evidences face, content, and ecological validity. Specifically, the tool was found to be truthful to established OM constructs, cover the full range of each OM constructs' meaning, and be feasible to use. Each of these areas is discussed with evidence and examples from the transcripts. In addition, we present practitioners' discussions of the usefulness of standardized information gathering techniques in the study of OM.

MA4-4

Patient satisfaction and perceived effectiveness on traditional Chinese medicine and western medicine: A population based comparative study

Chung V, Lau J, Wong E, Woo J, Lo SV, Griffiths S

School of Public Health, Chinese University of Hong Kong

Objective: The role of traditional Chinese medicine (TCM) as a part of the Hong Kong health care system was not formally recognized until the handover of the city's sovereignty from UK to mainland China in 1997. Population representative data collected as a Thematic Household Survey (THS) 2005 provided the first large scale cross sectional, comparative study of patient satisfaction and perceived effectiveness on TCM and western outpatient services. **Methods:** Face to face data collection interviews were conducted with 36,724 non-institutional and institutional residents, representing 6,504,255 persons after applying population weights. A subset of respondents who visited outpatient medical care in 30 days prior enumeration (western medical care (WM), n=5,953, and TCM care (TCM), n=810) were asked to assess the satisfaction of their latest consultations using a four questions selected from the NHS Local Health Services (NHS LHS) Questionnaire (Listening, respecting, timing, and explaining satisfactorily) and one on self perceived effectiveness of care. **Results:** With four being the best scoring for each question, the mean scores and their associated 95% CI for all five questions were higher than three in both TCM and WM group. However the mean scores for TCM care were higher than that of WM in all questions (Mann Whitney test, p< 0.05). For WM group, multiple logistic regression models for the four NHS LHS questions showed that respondents with self reported chronic disease were more likely to express dissatisfactions. Similar findings were not found in the TCM group. In contrast, older clients were more likely to rate favorably on the listening skills of both TCM and WM providers. For TCM group, respondents with primary or tertiary education level were more likely to be satisfied with the respect expressed by their TCM practitioners. Logistic models for self perceived effectiveness questions suggested that older respondents were more likely to score higher, in both TCM and WM care. **Conclusion:** This is the first population based study comparing the patient satisfaction and perceived effectiveness on TCM and WM care in Hong Kong and two important findings were noted. Firstly, respondents were equally satisfied with the care provided by both TCM and WM practitioners in terms of satisfaction and perceived effectiveness, despite formal regulation and professional training for TCM were in place for less than 10 years. Secondly, TCM users tend to rate higher compared WM users, and chronic disease patients sought WM care were more likely to be dissatisfied. Therefore we hypothesise that the popularity of TCM amongst chronic disease patients in Hong Kong, as suggested by previous studies, is linked to higher satisfaction. This presentation will discuss the issues raised and suggest areas for future research.

MA4-5

Effectiveness of Gua Sha in chronic neck pain: Results of a randomized controlled clinical trial

Schwickert M, Braun M, Lüdtke R, Michalsen A, Musial F, Dobos G

Chair of Complementary Medicine, University of Duisburg-Essen; Department of Internal and Integrative Medicine, Kliniken Essen-Mitte, Germany

Aims: Gua Sha, therapeutic surface frictioning that intentionally raises petechiae, is a traditional East Asian healing technique. We aimed to examine whether a single Gua Sha treatment can reduce pain and improve function in patients with chronic neck pain more than a common control treatment. **Methods:** Patients (age 19–70) with chronic neck pain and an initial VAS pain score >3 cm were eligible. Major exclusion criteria were skin diseases, hemophilic disorders, invasive treatment of the cervical spine or pertinent soft tissue, rheumatic diseases, or treatment with anticoagulants. Patients were randomised into verum or control group and followed up for 7 days. 24 verum patients were treated with a single Gua Sha massage in the region of upper back/neck. 24 control patients were treated with a single local application of a ginger heat pad. The primary outcome measure was pain one week after treatment, assessed with VAS. Secondary outcomes were pain related to movement, pain at other time points, scores on the neck disability index (NDI) and the SF-36. **Results:** The primary outcome measure showed a statistically significant difference in VAS score in favour of GuaSha (group difference -22.9 cm, 95%-CI: -43.3 to -16.6 cm, p=0.0003, multiple ANCOVA) between the 2 study groups. From the secondary outcome measures, the NDI-score and the physical function and general health items of the SF-36 showed statistically significant differences in favour of Gua Sha. **Conclusions:** Gua Sha seems to have a beneficial short term effect on pain and functional status in patients with chronic neck pain. Acknowledgements: The study was funded by the Karl and Veronica Carstens Foundation, Essen, Germany.

MA5-1

Is honey an effective and safe treatment for venous leg ulcers? Findings from the HALT (honey as adjuvant therapy for leg ulcers) trial

Walker N, Jull A, Parag V, Molan P, Arroll B, Waters J, Latta A, Betts J, McAuley S, Hammond C, Rodgers A

Clinical Trials Research Unit, University of Auckland, New Zealand

Aim: The effectiveness of honey as a treatment for venous leg ulcers has not been evaluated despite widespread practitioner and lay interest in its use. The HALT trial (ISRCTN 06161544) aimed to evaluate the safety and efficacy of manuka honey in healing venous leg ulcers. **Methods:** Study design: Open label, multi-centre, randomised trial. Setting: Auckland, Waikato and Christchurch regions of New Zealand. Study population: People with venous leg ulcers currently under the care of district nursing services. Study treatments: Participants were allocated to calcium alginate dressing impregnated with manuka honey or usual care (dressing of clinician's choice). All participants received compression bandaging. Primary outcome: The proportion of participants healed at 12 weeks. Secondary outcomes: Time to healing, change in ulcer area, incidence of wound infection, costs per healed ulcer, adverse events, and health-related quality of life. Sample size: 400 people (200 in each group) will provide 90% power at p=0.05 to detect a 30% relative increase in the proportion completely healed at 12 weeks. Analyses: Intention-to-treat used. Incidence rates, relative risks and 95% confidence intervals (CI) were obtained for binary variables, with multiple logistic regression analysis conducted if confounding existed. Continuous data were analysed using Cox regression modelling. **Results:** A total of 368 people were randomised in the trial, with 362 participants (98%) followed up at 12 weeks. 104 (55.6%) participants in the honey-treated group and 90 (49.7%) in the usual care group healed at 12 weeks (absolute increase 5.9%, 95% CI -4.3% to 16.1%). Time to healing, change in ulcer area, incidence of infection, quality of life, and cost were not significantly different between the groups. Only minor adverse events were reported, with significantly fewer events occurring in the usual care group (relative risk 1.3, 95% CI 1.1 to 1.6). **Conclusions:** Honey-impregnated dressings do not confer substantial benefit in healing venous leg ulcers. HALT is an excellent example of how a clinical trial design can effectively evaluate an alternative therapy, and how a well-designed trial in the CAM area can obtain competitive public funding.

MA5-2

Supplementary treatment with the extract of Agaricus Blazei Murill improves insulin resistance in type 2 diabetes: A randomized, double-blind and placebo-controlled clinical trial

Hsu CH[1,4], Hwang KC[2], Liao YL[3], Lin SC[3], Chou P[4]

[1]Department of Chinese Medicine, Taipei Hospital, Taiwan; [2]Department of Pediatrics, Taipei Hospital, Taiwan; [3]Department of Endocrinology, Taipei Hospital, Taiwan; [4]The Community Medicine Research Center and Institute of Public Health, National Yang-Ming University, Taipei, Taiwan

Background: Complementary and alternative medicine use in Type 2 diabetic adults is popular. This study is to determine whether the supplement of Mushroom Agaricus Blazei Murill (ABM) extract improves insulin resistance in Type 2 diabetes. **Methods:** This study was a clinical randomized double-blind placebo-controlled trial. Of a population of 536 registered diabetes patients, 72 subjects (1) aged between 30 and 75 years, (2) being Chinese, (3) having Type 2 diabetes for more than one year, and (4) having been taking gliclazide and metformin for more than 6 months were enrolled in this study. The enrolled patients were randomly assigned to either receiving supplement of ABM extract or placebo (cellulose) 1500 gm daily for 12 weeks. Homeostasis model assessment for insulin resistance (HOMA-IR) was used as the major outcome measurement. **Results:** At the end of the study, subjects who received supplement of ABM extract (n = 29) showed significantly lower HOMA-IR index (3.6±2.5 vs 6.6±7.4; p = 0.04) than the control group (n = 31). The plasma adiponectin concentration increased 20.0(40.7) % in the ABM group after 12 weeks of treatment, but decreased in placebo group. **Conclusion:** Supplement of ABM extract improves insulin resistance among Type 2 diabetes subjects. The increase in adiponectin concentration after taking AMB extract for 12 weeks might be the mechanism that brings the beneficial effect. Studies with longer period of follow-up should be conducted in the future.

MA5-3

The TU-025 Keishi Bukuryo Gan clinical trial for hot flash management: Outcomes, lessons and next steps

Plotnikoff GA[1,2], Radosevich D[2], LaValleur J[2], Torkelson C[2], Watanabe K[1]

[1]Keio University School of Medicine, Tokyo, Japan; [2]University of Minnesota Medical School, Minneapolis, Minnesota, USA

Aims: TU025, a traditional Japanese herbal medicine which consists of four herbs and a mushroom, successfully treats post-menopausal hot flashes in Japanese women. This study assessed TU025's potential efficacy in American women. **Methods:** This randomized, double-blind, placebo-controlled, phase II trial enrolled 175 post-menopausal women, aged 45-58 years, with a hot flash score of greater than 28 per week and who met other inclusion criteria. After a one-week placebo run-in period, subjects were randomly assigned to one of three arms (placebo, 7.5 g/day or 12.5 g/day) for the 12 week trial. The Mayo Clinic Hot Flash Diary documented the frequency and severity of hot flashes. Sleep quality was assessed by the Pittsburgh Sleep Quality Index (PSQI) and depression, somatic and vasomotor symptoms were assessed by the Greene Climacteric Index (GCI). Data were analyzed using mixed model and generalized estimating equations (GEE) methods with the last value carried forward for missing values. The outcomes in the two intervention groups were compared with the placebo group. **Results:** At three months, hot flash scores decreased by 34% in the placebo group, 40% in the 7.5 g/day group and 38% in the 12.5 g/day group. These declines in mean scores were significant (p<0.001). However, the differences between groups were not statistically significant (p=0.99). There was a trend ($p<0.1$) toward greater reduction of hot flashes in lean women ($p=0.09$), women with low estradiol levels ($p=0.062$) and women without hysterectomies ($p=0.067$). Simultaneous adjustment for all three variables approached statistical significance ($p=0.032$) after Bonferroni adjustment. Improvement in climacteric symptoms and sleep quality was documented across all three arms ($p<0.001$). Comparison across treatment conditions was not statistically significant. Diarrhea was present in 20% of participants receiving TU025. **Conclusions:** For post-menopausal American women, this study failed to confirm the capacity of TU025 to reduce the frequency and severity of hot flashes symptoms, improve climacteric symptoms or benefit sleep quality. Separate subgroup analysis suggests efficacy in a subpopulation of women closer to post-menopausal Japanese women. A follow up phase II trial is planned to further assess both traditional Asian and classical Western inclusion/exclusion criteria.

MA5-4

How well does Kampo, traditional Japanese herbal medicine, meet FDA requirements for clinical research?

Watanabe K, Plotnikoff GA

Department of Kampo Medicine, Keio University School of Medicine, Tokyo, Japan

Aims: To describe the extent that prescription Kampo formulas, traditional Japanese herbal medicines, qualify for United States Food and Drug Administration (FDA) Investigational New Drug Status (IND) and therefore rapid approval by Institutional Review Boards (IRB). **Methods:** The FDA's Center for Drug Evaluation and Research (CDER) publication, "Guidance for Industry: Botanical Drug Products" was reviewed and its standards were analyzed for applicability to phase I and phase II trials of ancient, multi-herb Asian formulas. **Results:** Because Kampo medicine is already used in Japan as a prescription drug, it belongs to the category of "INDs for phase 1 and phase 2 clinical studies of lawfully marketed botanical products without safety concerns". This requires 1) Description of the investigational product and documentation of the historical experience of human use, 2) Chemistry, Manufacturing and Controls, 3) Pharmacology/Toxicology Information. Because more than 30 years of pre-clinical research data already exists on Kampo formulas, and because of Japan's pharmaceutical grade production standards and prescription drug post-marketing surveillance program, most of the FDA requirements are easy to meet. Challenges common to all ancient multi-herb formulas are the absence of single active components and the absence of pharmacodynamic data. The probable presence of multiple but unidentified active components in extremely small concentrations undermines the capacity to determine precise dosing guidelines. Currently, three Kampo formulas have IND approvals for clinical study in the US including TU025 Keishi Bukuryo Gan. **Conclusion:** Prescription Kampo herbal medicines, perhaps more easily than any other traditional Asian medicine, meet the requirements for IND applications to the FDA. Kampo medicines may represent the best traditional Asian medicines for clinical trials in the United States and Europe.

MA5-5

Hawthorn extract does not inhibit clinical progression in patients with mild to moderate symptoms of heart failure

Zick S, Aaronson K

Department of Family Medicine, University of Michigan, USA

Background: Hawthorn (Crataegus monogyna) leaves, flowers and berries have been used to treat heart disease for at least 500 years. We tested the hypothesis that hawthorn extract (Crataegus Special Extract WS 1442, Crataegutt® forte) inhibits clinical progression in patients with NYHA II and III symptomatic heart failure due to left ventricular (LV) systolic dysfunction. **Methods:** We performed a secondary data analysis of a randomized, double blind, placebo controlled trial of a hawthorn extract in patients (n=120) with mild to moderate symptomatic heart failure, LV ejection fraction (LVEF) 0.40. Subjects had moderate functional impairment (defined as the ability to walk 150 to 450 m on a 6-minute walk test) and were receiving optimal standard therapy including ACE inhibitors, diuretics and beta blockers. Subjects were randomized to either hawthorn extract, WS 1442, 450 mg bid (n=60) or placebo (n=60) and followed up for 6 months in the HERB CHF trial. The main endpoint of the analysis was time to progression of heart failure, defined as death due to heart failure, hospitalization for heart failure, or a sustained increase in diuretic medications used for heart failure, as assessed by Kaplan-Meier analysis and Cox modeling, adjusting for potentially important prognostic determinants (age, gender, heart failure etiology, creatinine, NYHA functional class, serum sodium, peak oxygen consumption, LVEF, mean blood pressure, Heart Failure Survival Score, beta blocker and ACE inhibitor use). **Results:** Time to progression of heart failure occurred 14% earlier in the hawthorn group compared to the placebo group, although this was non-significant (hazard ratio 1.14; CI 0.60 to 2.15, $p=0.69$). Clinical progression of heart failure occurred in 32% of placebo patients and 32% of hawthorn patients, reflecting no ($p=1.00$) reduction in the secondary end point of heart failure progression (relative risk, 1.00; CI 0.46 to 2.16). The effect of hawthorn extract on time to heart failure progression was not influenced by any of the prognostic determinants examined. **Conclusions:** Hawthorn extract, when added to standard therapy does not reduce clinical progression in patients who have mild to moderate symptomatic heart failure.

MA6-1

Efficacy of a hypnotic relaxation intervention as adjunct to analgesic medication for women who are undergoing a first trimester pregnancy termination: An open non-inferiority trial

Marc I, Rainville P, Vallée E, Verreault R, Vaillancourt L, Masse B, Dodin S

Lucie et André Chagnon Chair's for the teaching of an integrated approach in prevention, Laval University

Background: To provide additional control of pain, a wide range of medications has been offered to the women during surgery abortion procedure but efficacy of intravenous conscious sedation and oral medications on pain and anxiety control does not completely encounter patient's satisfaction. The purpose of this study was to generate evidence to enable health professionals to consider the role of non pharmacological approaches to manage gynecologic procedural pain in women. **Methods:** We did an open randomized clinical trial in one center at the Family planning clinic of Hôpital Saint-François d'Assise (CHUQ), Université Laval (Quebec City, Canada). 350 women undergoing surgical abortion were randomly assigned to receive either standard care or in addition to standard care, a hypnotic relaxation intervention including analgesia suggestions 20 minutes before and throughout the surgical procedure. Patients in both groups were given the option to control their pain by intravenous sedation that was standardized to 75 ug of fentanyl and 2 mg of midazolam. The primary outcome was to determine whether a hypnotic relaxation intervention could modify the request of intravenous conscious sedation during the surgical abortion procedure while not being inferior in terms of patient's anxiety and pain intensity level. **Results:** 108/172 (63%) of the women assigned to the hypnotic relaxation intervention had received sedation (fentanyl and midazolam) during the procedure versus 149/175 (85%) of the women assigned to the standard care group ($p<0.0001$). No differences were found between the groups in self-reports of pain and anxiety by the women at the most painful step of the surgery (suction-evacuation). **Discussion:** In the clinical management of abdominal pain during surgery for abortion, a short hypnotic relaxation intervention is well accepted by the women. Such intervention can safely decrease the request of IV sedation (fentanyl and midazolam) by the women by around 20% without increasing their levels of pain and anxiety during the procedure.

MA6-2

A controlled trial to compare three treatment options for patients suspecting health complaints due to dental amalgam

Melchart D[1,2], Vogt S[3], Köhler W[1], Streng A[1], Weidenhammer W[1], Kremers L[3], Hickel R[3], Felgenhauer N[4], Zilker T[4], Wühr E[5], Halbach S[6]

[1]Centre for Complementary Medicine Research, Technical University Munich, Germany; [2]Division of Complementary Medicine, University Hospital Zurich, Switzerland; [3]Department of Restorative Dentistry, Periodontology and Pediatric Dentistry, University of Munich; [4]Department of Clinical Toxicology, Internal Medicine II, Technical University Munich; [5]International Association for Holistic Dental Medicine, Mannheim, Germany; [6]Institute of Toxicology, GSF Research Centre for Environment and Health, Munich

Background: Some bearers of dental amalgam with chronic, non-specific health problems suspect that their complaints are due to mercury release from their fillings. Evidence from prospective trials is scarce which treatment should be recommended. **Aim:** To compare reduction of subjective complaints by three treatment strategies in so called 'amalgam patients' whose complaints could not be explained by a medical or psychological disorder. **Methods:** 90 patients complying with predefined inclusion and exclusion criteria were randomly assigned either to removal of dental amalgam only (group A), or removal in combination with a 'biological detoxification' therapy with high doses of vitamins and trace elements (group B), or participation in a health promotion program without removal of dental amalgam (group C). Outcome measurements were the decrease in a weighted sum score (0 to 10 points) of main complaints from baseline to month 12 (main outcome), and change in psychometric questionnaires and in mercury levels in blood and urine. **Results:** With regard to the main outcome measure, group A improved by 3.5 (2.2) (mean, SD) points from a baseline of 6.9 (1.1), group B by 3.5 (2.2) from a baseline of 7.4 (1.0) and group C by 2.5 (2.4) from a baseline of 7.3 (0.8). Difference between groups was not statistically significant. Amalgam removal in groups A and B was associated with a significant decrease in steady state levels of inorganic mercury and clinically relevant improvements in subjective health complaints. Group C showed similar improvements in subjective complaints, although mercury levels deviated only slightly from baseline. **Conclusions:** 'Amalgam patients' will benefit from suitable therapy, but such therapy is not limited to the removal of amalgam.

MA6-3

Application of multi-site ultra-weak photon emission recording in practitioners of meditation programs

Van Wijk EPA[1], Van Wijk R[1,2]

[1]International Institute of Biophysics, Neuss, Germany;
[2]Faculty of Biology, Utrecht University, The Netherlands

Aims: The reduction of stress claimed to result from meditation may have prophylactic and therapeutic health benefits. An interesting hypothesis has been raised regarding a possible link between meditation and its therapeutic effect utilizing recent information about the contribution of oxidative stress to the physiology of arteriosclerosis, coronary heart disease, and other chronic diseases. Therefore, it might be productive to investigate the influence of meditation on free radical mediated oxidation processes, utilizing modern physical technology recording spontaneous ultra-weak photon emission (UPE) non-invasively from multiple body locations. **Methods:** The study examined the anatomical pattern of UPE of 20 subjects practicing transcendental meditation (TM) compared to 20 subjects who were practicing other meditation techniques (OTM) and 20 control subjects without experience in meditation. Subjects were men reported to be healthy and non-smokers. UPE was recorded in a dark room using a highly sensitive, cooled photomultiplier system designed for manipulation in three directions. The protocol for multi-site registration of UPE includes recording of 12 anatomic locations of anterior torso, head, neck and hands. **Results:** Data demonstrate emission intensities in the TM group and OTM group that are 27 and 17 percent lower, respectively, compared to the control group. All subjects demonstrated a "common" anatomic pattern of UPE. The percent emission contribution of each location to total emission was very similar for the three groups. The differences in emission could not be ascribed to age differences. **Conclusions:** Data support the conclusion that life styles including persistent meditation resulted in a decrease of oxidative stress. The present study also demonstrated that TM techniques resulted in the largest effect.

MA6-4

Expectancy in treatment of metabolic syndrome and obesity

Calabrese C[1], Tippens K[1], Connelly E[1], Purnell J[2]

[1]Helfgott Research Institute at the National College of Natural Medicine (NCNM), [2]Oregon Health and Science University, USA

This on-going pilot study explores effects of expectancies associated with different clinical trial designs for a dietary supplement in a 3-arm 12-week trial of 90 overweight men and women with metabolic syndrome. The placebo effect of an oral agent is used as a model of patient expectancy in this study. The study's specific aims are to 1) determine if there is detectable enhancement of weight loss with a placebo; 2) gather data on the locus of impact by group on perception, behavior, and chemistry measures; 3) characterize differences between placebo-responders and non-responders. Participants were eligible for the study if obese (BMI>30) and having metabolic syndrome, i.e., having 3 or more of 5 criteria: high blood pressure, high fasting blood glucose, high triglycerides, low HDL cholesterol, and a waist circumference over 35 inches for women and 40 inches for men. All subjects received education for diet and exercise. Subjects in one arm were given a placebo and told they were in a placebo-controlled randomized double-blinded trial of an active agent where they could receive either the active or placebo supplement (50% expectancy of getting the active agent); in a second arm, subjects were given placebo and told that they were taking the active agent (100% expectancy); the third arm received only education (0% expectancy). Measures of differences between groups were anthropometric, psychometric, behavioral, metabolic and hormonal. Based on preliminary data, participants in both the 100% and 50% expectancy groups lost more weight and lowered BMI more than those in the 0% expectancy group, suggesting that placebo expectancy impacts weight loss (ANOVA $p < .05$) with the 50% expectancy group showing the greatest weight loss. Other measures will be analyzed at the completion of clinical activities.

MA6-5

Placebo treatment improves physical, but not biochemical outcome parameters of peripheral organ diseases

Meissner K, Distel H, Mitzdorf U

Institute of Medical Psychology, Ludwig-Maximilians University Munich, Germany

Aims: Evidence for placebo treatment to objectively improve peripheral disease processes is still scarce. We performed a review of placebo effects in clinical trials and hypothesized that at least a subset of peripheral outcome parameters would be responsive to placebo treatment. **Methods:** A first dataset was collected from a Medline search for placebo-controlled clinical trials. Trials with stable disease conditions were selected, and the effect of placebo treatment was estimated by changes from baseline in the placebo groups. Placebo effects on different types of parameters were examined in order to identify parameter classes with differential placebo responsiveness. The resulting classification was further established by performing an n-weighted subgroup meta-analysis of the placebo effects' standardized mean differences. A subgroup meta-analysis of a second dataset of clinical trials was added to test whether the preliminary classification would also apply to placebo effects derived from the comparison of placebo groups with untreated control groups. **Results:** The analysis of the first dataset suggested a classification into placebo-responsive "physical" versus placebo non-responsive "biochemical" parameters: 50% of trials measuring physical parameters showed significant placebo effects compared to 6% of trials measuring biochemical parameters. The subgroup meta-analysis substantiated the differential response (physical parameters: n=14, g=0.34, 95% CI 0.22 to 0.46; biochemical parameters: n=15, g=0.03, 95% CI -0.04 to 0.10). The subgroup meta-analysis of the second dataset further supported the classification; it revealed a significant improvement for physical parameters (n=20, g=0.22, 95% CI 0.07 to 0.36) and a deterioration for biochemical parameters (n=6, g=-0.17, 95% CI -0.31 to -0.02). **Conclusions:** The results suggest that placebo treatment can improve physical disease processes of peripheral organs more easily and strongly than biochemical ones. This differential response may best be explained by a mechanism of visceral reward learning, which may be accomplished only for disease processes providing contingent feedback to cortical areas involved in autonomic control.

MA7-1

Effects of a herbal formula modalities on bone density – a randomized, double-blind, placebo-controlled clinical trial

Leung PC, Cheng KF

Institute of Chinese Medicine, The Chinese University of Hong Kong, China

Background and aim: Bone loss leading to osteoporosis, which has its highest rate of occurrence in postmenopausal women, increases the risk for fractures. Osteoporosis can be prevented or limited by maximizing the bone strength and minimizing the bone mass loss. Traditional Chinese medicine (TCM) has been serving the people in China since over 2000 years ago and remains an important part of health care provision in modern China. The herbal formula containing mainly *Epimedium* was found to have some properties in the treatment and prevention of postmenopausal osteoporosis. The aim of the study was to determine the changes in bone material properties and the biomarkers of bone metabolism induced by the herbal formula treatment in post-menopausal women. **Method:** The study was designed as a single-center, prospective, randomized, double-blind, placebo-controlled study. Postmenopausal women aged 51 to 67 were randomized to Herbal capsule (n=75) or Placebo (n=75) by daily oral for 12 months. All subjects received daily oral supplement of 1000mg calcium. Hip femoral neck and spinal bone mineral density (BMD) was determined by dual-energy x-ray absorptiometry. The BMD was measured at baseline, 6- month and 12-month during the study period. Blood biochemical marker bone ALP for bone metabolism was also measured. The safety of the herbal capsule was investigated as well. **Results:** After 12 months hip femoral neck and spinal BMD increased compared to baseline (0.67% and 0.19%, respectively) in the TCM group, but decreased in the placebo group (-1.31% and -1.40%, respectivley). For subjects age less than 60 years old, hip femoral neck BMD was increased 1.71% compared with baseline (p=0.080) in the TCM group, while it decreased 2.52% in the placebo group. The average percent change in hip femoral neck BMD in the TCM group was higher than that in the placebo group (p=0.077). These results indicated that the study herbal capsule has effects of preventing bone loss in postmenopausal women. **Conclusions:** The study results imply that the herbal formula might delay the occurrence of bone loss.

MA7-2

A randomised placebo-controlled clinical trial of a Chinese herbal medicine for the treatment of vascular dementia

Liu J[1], Chang D[1], Chan D[2], Cordato D[2], Bensoussan A[1]

[1]Centre for Complementary Medicine Research, University of Western Sydney, Australia; [2]Bankstown-Lidcome Hospital, University of New South Wales, Australia

Background: Vascular dementia (VaD) is the second most common cause of dementia after Alzheimer's disease and accounts for 15-20 percent of all cases of dementia in Western countries. Chinese herbal medicine has been used for the treatment of dementia-like disorders for centuries. Although some data exists to support its use, strong scientific evidence is generally lacking. Wei Nao Kang (WNK) is a complex herbal formula that consists of the concentrated extracts of three Chinese herbs. The preclinical experiments of WNK have demonstrated statistically significant improvement in learning and memory function in dementia animal models. **Aims:** The aim of this study was to investigate the clinical effectiveness of WNK for the treatment of VaD. **Methods:** This is a randomized, double-blinded, and placebo-controlled clinical trial. The diagnosis of VaD was based on the National Institute for Neurologic Disease and Stroke and the Association Internationale pour la Recherche et l'Enseignement en Neurosciences (NINDS-AIREN) criteria. Patients received a 16 weeks double-blind treatment of active or identical placebo after randomization. Alzheimer's Disease Assessment Scale, cognitive sub-scale (ADAS-cog) was used as the primary efficacy parameter. Analyses were performed on an intention-to-treat basis. All the efficacy parameters were analyzed using T-test. **Results:** 62 patients with probable or possible VaD were recruited. ADAS-cog scores decreased significantly in patients receiving treatment with WNK compared to placebo ($p<0.01$). **Conclusion:** WNK appears to improve cognitive functions of the VaD patients and may be a useful alternative for the treatment of VaD.

MA7-3

The quality of reporting of randomized controlled trials in traditional Chinese medicine is improving but still in poor status

Wang G[1], Mao B[1], Xiong ZY[2], Fan T MD[1], Chen XD[3], Wang L[1], Liu GJ[4], Liu J[5], Guo J[1], Chang J[1], Wu TX[4], Li TQ[1]

[1]Department of Integrated Traditional Chinese and Western Medicine, West China Hospital, Sichuan University, Chengdu, China; [2]Department of Pharmacology, School of Medicine, Temple University, Philadelphia, USA; [3]West China School of Medicine, Sichuan University, Chengdu, China; [4]Chinese Cochrane Centre, West China Hospital, Sichuan University, Chengdu, China; [5]Chengdu University of Traditional Chinese Medicine, Chengdu, China

Background: The number of randomized controlled trials (RCTs) of traditional Chinese medicine (TCM) is increasing, but reviews before 1999 have shown that the quality of trials of TCM is very poor. **Objective:** To assess whether the quality of reporting of clinical trials in TCM is being improved. **Methods:** A retrospective survey. Setting: Chinese Cochrane centre and university department of TCM. Subjects and Measurements: 13 journals of TCM in mainland China were randomly selected, and all issues published from 1999 to 2004 were hand-searched according to the hand-search guideline of the Cochrane Centre. A comprehensive quality assessment of each RCT was completed using methods including the revised CONSORT checklist and Jadad scale. Disagreements were resolved by consensus. **Results:** The percentage of RCTs was significantly increased step by step, which was 18.6%, 23.9%, 27.5%, 28.7%, 33.0% and 35.6% from 1999 to 2004, and a total of 7422 RCTs were identified. 39.4% of the items in CONSORT, which is equivalent of 11.82 of a total of 30 items (SD=5.78), were reported across those trials. Furthermore, the mean Jadad score in all trials was 1.03±0.61, and the score was 0.85±0.53 (n=746), 0.82±0.63 (n=941), 0.90±0.61 (n=1243), 1.03±0.60 (n=1325), 1.12±0.58 (n=1533) and 1.20±0.62 (n=1634) from 1999 to 2004, which was improved continuously but slowly. **Conclusions** Estimates of trends for the quality of reporting of TCM RCTs were provided. Our findings suggest that important methodological components of TCM RCTs are incompletely reported, and key information unique to TCM trials may be missing, such as syndromes described in TCM, explanation of TCM rationale and quality assurance for herbs. An elaborated CONSORT statement for TCM seems desirable.

MA7-4

Placebo stick devices causing heat sensation are no valid sham control procedure for moxibustion

Pach D[1], Piazena H[2], Willich SN[1], Brinkhaus B[1]

[1]Institute for Social Medicine, Epidemiology, and Health Economics and [2]Clinic for Psychiatry and Psychotherapy, Charité University Medical Center, Berlin, Germany

Background: Moxa sticks are used in traditional Chinese medicine to stimulate acupuncture points with heat from the slow combustion of mugwort. There is no valid placebo method available for sham controlled randomized controlled trials to investigate the effectiveness of moxibustion. A convincing placebo moxa stick device should be capable of evoking heat sensation without a therapeutic effect. By measurement of the spectral infrared irradiance of seven different moxa sticks the potential of a placebo moxa stick device causing a heat sensation by emitting only epidermal affecting infrared radiation C (IR-C) was evaluated. **Methods:** An IR radiometer was used to measure the spectral infrared irradiance of seven glowing moxa sticks of different types in dependence of distance to the heat. **Results:** All sticks investigated show a similar spectral distribution of the emitted IR radiation with maxima of about 83.5% to 87.5% in the range long wavelength IR radiation (IR-C) and with small contributions of both short wavelength IR radiation (IR-A) between 2.2% to 5.5% and of middle wavelength IR radiation (IR-B) between 9.0% to 12.1% of the total IR emission. Differences in stick's characteristics resulted in differences of total irradiance at given distances of the heat up to a factor of about 3 between the thinnest and the thickest stick. **Conclusion:** Only a small proportion of the moxa stick's emitted IR radiation is capable of affecting subepidermal tissue. These results indicate that effects due to moxa sticks are caused by superficial effects on the skin. Since most heat receptors are located in the superficial skin, it seems impossible to separate effects from moxa stick from heat sensation. Therefore placebo stick devices causing heat sensation seem not suitable sham control therapies. Comparing moxa stick treatment with standard western treatment and waiting list group is an alternative option. Future clinical moxa studies should include descriptions of the physical characteristics of the applied moxa. Data on dose-effect ratio of moxa sticks is needed.

MA7-5

Factors associated with allocation guesses in the Acupuncture Randomized Trials (ART)

Linde K[1], Witt CW[2], Brinkhaus B[2], Streng A[1], Willich SN[2], Weidenhammer W[1], Melchart D[1]

[1]Center for Complementary Medicine Research, Technical University of Munich, Germany; [2]Institute for Social Medicine, Epidemiology, and Health Economics, Charité University Medical Center, Berlin, Germany

Background: Unblinding is a relevant potential problem in many controlled trials. In an increasing number of trials patients are asked at the end of the study to make a guess which treatment they think they have been allocated to. If guesses differ between groups this is interpreted as evidence for unblinding. However, apart from the actual treatment other factors such as the perceived effect and the course of the disease are likely to influence such guesses. We aimed to investigate factors associated with allocation guesses in four randomized trials of acupuncture. **Methods:** Data of all 864 patients allocated to acupuncture or minimal acupuncture (superficial needling at non-acupuncture points) in the Acupuncture Randomized Trials (ART) on migraine, tension-type headache, chronic low back pain and osteoarthritis of the knee were pooled. All patients had been asked at the end of the trials to make a guess of treatment allocation. Multiple logistic regression analyses were performed to investigate which factors were associated with specific guesses about allocation. **Results:** In the migraine trial which had shown no difference between acupuncture and minimal acupuncture allocation guesses differed strongly between groups ($p < 0.001$) while in the trial on osteoarthritis of the knee guesses were similar ($p = 0.33$) although this study had shown a superiority of "true" acupuncture after two months of treatment. In the two other trials allocation guesses differed to a moderate extent between the groups ($p = 0.04$ in the low back pain and 0.07 in the tension-type headache trial). In the multivariate analyses of the pooled data the guess "acupuncture" was significantly associated with an allocation to this group and a symptom improvement of at least 50%. The guess "minimal acupuncture" was significantly more frequent in patients allocated to this group and significantly less frequent in older patients and in patients suffering from osteoarthritis of the knee. **Conclusions:** The results of our pooled analyses suggest that the reasons why patients make specific guesses about treatment allocation at the end of a study are complex.

MA8-1

The MRC ATEAM trial of Alexander technique, exercise and massage for chronic and recurrent back pain: Is there hope for chronic back pain sufferers?

Little P[1], Webley F[1], Beattie A[4], Evans M[4], Middelton K[1], Barnett J[1], Lewith G[1], Ballard K[5], Oxford F[5], Smith P[2], Yardley L[3], Hollingshurst S[4], Sharp D[4]

[1]Primary Care group, CCS Division, University of Southampton, UK; [2]Department of Social Statistics, University of Southampton, UK; [3]School of Psychology, University of Southampton, UK; [4]Primary Care group, University of Bristol, UK; [5]The Society of Teachers of the Alexander Technique, UK

Context: Chronic back pain is a major problem for patients, health care providers, and society but there are very few proven interventions. **Objective:** To assess the effectiveness of massage, a physical activity prescription, and the Alexander Technique (a self-care approach that facilitates avoidance of pain-producing misuse and the re-establishment of normal neuro-muscular co-ordination) for back pain. **Design:** Randomised controlled trial. **Setting:** Primary care. **Patients:** 579 patients with chronic or recurrent back pain. **Intervention:** Four groups: normal care (control); 6 sessions of massage; 6 lessons of Alexander Technique (6AT); and 24 lessons of Alexander Technique (24AT). Half of each of these groups was also randomised to GP exercise prescription with follow-up behavioural counselling sessions from the practice nurse. **Results:** At 3 months all interventions improved the Roland Morris (RM) function score (the main outcome). By 1 year the effect of massage was no longer significant, but the effect of Alexander Technique was maintained (mean reduction in RM score compared to the control group: massage -0.58 (95% confidence intervals -1.94 to 0.77); 6AT -1.40 (-2.77 to -0.03); 24AT -3.4 (-4.76; -2.03). Exercise was also effective (-1.29 (-2.25 to -0.34)). Exercise combined with 6AT achieved 71% of the impact of Exercise and 24AT (RM score respectively -2.98 (-4.99 to -1.07) and -4.22 (-6.13 to -2.31)). At 1 year the median number of days of back pain reported in the last 4 weeks was much lower with Alexander Technique: control 21 days, massage 15 days, 6AT 10 days, and 24AT 3 days. Alexander Technique also improved quality of life, and both exercise and Alexander Technique reduced fear avoidance (fear of harm due to physical activity). **Conclusion:** The Alexander Technique has a major long term effect on both pain and function, and improves quality of life for patients with chronic or recurrent back pain. A short course of Alexander Technique lessons combined with exercise prescription is nearly as effective as a longer course of lessons and could feasibly be considered by health care providers.

MA8-2

Patients perceptions and satisfaction with treatment in a UK osteopathic training clinic

Leach CMJ[1], Strutt R[2], Shaw Q[2]

[1]Clinical Research Centre for Health Professions, University of Brighton, UK; [2]Surrey Institute of Osteopathic Medicine, North East Surrey College of Technology, Ewell, UK

This study was a descriptive and exploratory investigation of patient perceptions of treatment at an osteopathic training clinic. The primary aim was to understand the factors contributing to patient satisfaction and dissatisfaction, and to understand patients' perceptions of care, outcomes and quality of their treatment. A semi-structured questionnaire survey was administered by post in 2000 to all 292 patients attending the clinic 1998-2000. The response rate was 62%. The data comprised free text, which was transcribed and analysed in stages. A content analysis showed that over 90% of subjects reported being satisfied or highly satisfied with treatment, and 76% respondents perceived that their health had improved as a result of treatment. The concepts within the data were coded using grounded theory, within an interpretive phenomenological approach. "Patient centred" emerged as the core theme, associated with the four main themes of Hope, Communication, Respect, and Trust. Two further themes were interwoven throughout the comments: firstly, issues related to being seen at a Teaching Clinic and, secondly, Cross-Checking of the standards and quality of care in this clinic against others, particularly the NHS, but also other complementary and musculoskeletal therapies and other osteopathic clinics. The survey elicited some strong emotions from a few patients: embarrassment about undressing and anger about perceived lack of privacy during treatment. The study has implications for service delivery in both student training clinics and private practice. Recommendations are made for the design of future studies in this area.

MA8-3

The effects of reflexology on pain threshold and tolerance in an ice-pain experiment in healthy human subjects

Samuel CA, Ebenezer IS

Department of Pharmacy and Biomedical Sciences, University of Portsmouth, UK

Background: Reflexology incorporates the use of specific pressure techniques to the feet, hands or ears. It has been claimed that reflexology is useful in the treatment of various conditions including such things as migraine, arthritis and multiple sclerosis. The aim of the present study was to investigate whether foot reflexology attenuates acute pain in human volunteers. **Methods:** Ten healthy male (n=4) and female (n=6) subjects were each assigned to single treatments of both reflexology and sham TENS (transcutaneous electrical nerve stimulation; Control) administered in a cross-over design. Pain was induced in both treatment schemes by immersion of the non-dominant hand in crushed ice (1). Two measurements were taken (i) pain threshold (i.e. the time it takes for the subject to find the experience painful) and (ii) pain tolerance (i.e. the time it takes until the subject can no longer keep his/her hand in the ice water). Measurements were taken 15 mins prior to treatment and at 30 min intervals for 120 mins following reflexology or sham TENS. The data were analysed by two-way analysis of variance (ANOVA) with repeated measures on treatment and time and the Dunnett's post-hoc test. **Results:** ANOVA showed that there was a significant increase in pain threshold of the subjects following reflexology when compared with sham TENS control data ($F(1,9)=5.68$, $p<0.05$). Thus, for example at 60 min, pain threshold increased from a control mean value (sham TENS) ± s.e. mean of 9.1±1.4s to 15.5±2.1s following reflexology ($p<0.01$). Similarly, there was a significant increase in pain tolerance ($F(1,9) = 5.132$, $p<0.05$). Thus, at 60 min, pain tolerance increased from a control mean value ± s.e. mean of 120.2±37.9s to 171.4±42.0s ($p<0.02$). **Conclusion:** The results of this study show that reflexology increases both pain threshold and tolerance in human volunteers exposed to acute pain. These findings indicate the possibility of using reflexology in the management of pain.

MA8-4

Fascia is able to contract and relax in a smooth muscle-like manner and thus may influence musculoskeletal dynamics

Schleip R[1], Zorn A[1], Lehmann-Horn F[1], Klingler W[2]

[1]Fascia Research Project, Institute of Applied Physiology, Ulm University, Germany; [2]Department of Anesthesiology, Ulm University, Germany

Aims: Clinical observations from osteopaths and acupuncturists suggest that fascia may be able to autonomously change its stiffness. This study examined the hypothesis that fascia – due to the presence of smooth muscle-like fibroblasts (myofibroblasts) – can actively contract and thereby influence musculoskeletal dynamics. **Methods:** An immunohistochemical analysis was performed, focusing on the monoclonal myofibroblast marker alpha-smooth muscle actin, using tissue samples of lumbodorsal fascia, plantar fascia and fascia lata from 32 human bodies. Additionally mechanographic force measurements were conducted using strips of fresh rat lumbodorsal fascia and human fascia lata. Force differences between maximal tissue contraction and relaxation were hypothetically calculated for the cross sectional area of all lumbar fasciae at the level of L4/L5 in an average human body. **Results:** Immunohistochemistry: Myofibroblasts were present in all tissues. Their density in the lumbodorsal fascia was significantly higher than in plantar fascia or fascia lata ($p<0.05$). Mechanographic tests were performed in an organ bath under isometric strain, checking the response to pharmacological stimulation. Stimulation with the myofibroblast agonist mepyramine elicited active tissue contractions lasting up to 2hrs. Stimulation with the smooth muscle relaxant glyceryl trinitrate induced relaxation. Unviable control tissues did not react, indicating that a cellular mechanism caused the response. The maximal observed force difference ($3.6mN/mm^2$) if applied to the human lumbar area would predict a total contraction force of >5N. **Conclusion:** Fascia is populated by myofibroblasts and is therefore able to actively contract and relax over a period of minutes or hours. This capacity seems to be especially expressed in human lumbodorsal fascia. The potential tonus changes in fascia are strong enough to be palpable and to impact musculoskeletal dynamics; such as through gamma motor regulation. This may have interesting implications for fascia-directed therapies like acupuncture, osteopathy, or Rolfing myofascial release.

MA8-5

Effects and experiences of Shiatsu: Results from a longitudinal, three country, cross-European study

Long AF

School of Healthcare, University of Leeds, UK

Introduction and Aims: While there is an increasing research base for energy therapies such as acupuncture, the research base on the client experiences and effects of shiatsu, a therapy whose philosophical underpinnings are similar to acupuncture, is limited. This paper reports on the emerging findings of a three-country, cross-European, longitudinal study aiming to map the characteristics of shiatsu receivers and to assess their experience and perceptions of short and longer-term, positive and negative, effects of shiatsu. **Methods:** Study Design: A longitudinal cohort study, undertaken in Austria, Spain and the UK Funder: European Shiatsu Federation. Client recruitment: Participating shiatsu practitioners, meeting two eligibility criteria (seeing ≥ 20 clients per month; on the national society's register since July 2003), followed a uniform research protocol to recruit sequentially up to 16, new and/or continuing clients. Data Collection: Four self-administered questionnaires completed by the client, at baseline recruitment, 4–7 days after the initial shiatsu session, 3 and 6 months later. The instruments were professionally translated and checked by native language speakers. Data collection is to be completed by April 2007. Data Analysis: Descriptive and analytical statistics, including t test, chi-square test and tests for trend; thematic analysis for verbatim comments. **Results:** To date, 935 clients have been recruited (366 Austria; 181 Spain; 388 UK) and 636, 3-month follow-up questionnaires returned (response rate of 68%). At baseline, the most common reasons for seeking treatment were 'out of curiosity', to maintain/improve health and/or to 'do something for oneself'. Common hopes from shiatsu were to relax, enhance energy and alleviate ill-health symptoms. Immediate effects, 7-days or so later, included feeling relaxed and 'energy or blockages moving'. About 25% had experienced a self-perceived minor negative, but transitional, effect. High levels of satisfaction and met expectations were evident. Three and six month data are still being collected. **Conclusion:** The study extends the evidence base on the experience and effects of shiatsu on health and well-being, providing the basis to explore the relative effectiveness of shiatsu to other CAM modalities and/or conventional medicine.

MA9-1

Healing and effect of CAM as hybrid phenomena

Johannessen H

Institute of Public Health, Research Unit Healt, Man and Society, University of Southern Denmark, Denmark

Based on experiences from a current cross-disciplinary team of researchers exploring effects of CAM for cancer through an application of methods from a variety of disciplines (oncology, nursing, psychology, economy and anthropology) this paper explores the feasibility of addressing the question of effects of CAM within the conceptual framework of hybrid actor networks as developed by Bruno Latour. Among the questions to be addressed is (1) the identification of healing as expressed by the patients and as a hybrid phenomena crossing the borders of natural science, social science and the humanities; (2) the identification of relevant effect parameters provided by the various disciplines involved in the research team; and (3) an exploration of research designs and methodologies that can encompass these effect parameters and their mutual connectedness in one common framework. The presentation is a suggestion for a conceptual frame for CAM-research and the aim is to open for a discussion with participants of the conference on how we can conceptualize and measure the effects of CAM in a way that recognizes the various effects experienced by the patients within a coherent and common multi-disciplinary scientific framework.

MA9-2

Developing patient-centered measures for outcomes of CAM therapies

Ritenbaugh C, Koithan M, Coons S, Verhoef M, Sutherland E, Warber S, Elder C

University of Arizona, Tucson, Arizona, USA

Many systems within complementary and alternative medicine (CAM) target the whole person and restoration of balance. There is evidence that some individuals receiving CAM therapies, especially therapies that might be considered to have an energetic or spiritual component, report what have been called transformative experiences - life-altering changes that transcend original symptoms. These experiences have often been lumped with "non-specific outcomes", and yet they may be specific to some types of CAM therapies. To date, researchers report few empirical studies of whole person-centered outcomes, as experienced by clients receiving either CAM or conventional therapies, to guide the choice of outcomes for evaluation. Reliable and valid tools are not available to evaluate the whole person-level and transformative experiences reported in qualitative interviews from a variety of studies. This project combines qualitative data collected in peer-reviewed research at five US and Canadian institutions to develop and subsequently evaluate an outcomes instrument that would have broad applicability in CAM research and potentially in conventional biomedical research as well. The overall goal is to develop and complete the psychometric evaluation of a questionnaire for use in CAM research to measure whole-person outcomes including transformational change. Here, we report on the first phase of this process, which will involve developing a draft data collection instrument based on the language of patients. The data source is qualitative interviews collected as part of seven different peer-reviewed research projects involving patients receiving CAM therapies. Researchers performed secondary analysis on patient (n=122) and practitioner (n=55) reports of changes experienced through CAM therapies. First, transcripts with content clearly relating to transformative experiences were selected (n=78). Transcript segments were coded using ATLAS Ti, a qualitative data analysis program. Particular attention was paid to participants' natural language of their experiences and descriptors of transformational changes. Items were chosen based on their consistency of usage and frequent appearance. The resulting draft instrument will be rigorously evaluated over the next two years in a variety of populations and CAM treatment settings. This project is supported by NCCAM grant R01AT003314.

MA9-3

Research literacy for complementary and alternative health care practitioners (CAHC) – an online course

Dryden T[1], Achilles R[2], Baskwill A[3], Finch P[4], Humphreys K[5], Kelner M[2], Leverkus G[6], Luke R[2], Mior S[7], Tailor-Vaisey A[8]

[1]Applied Research Centre, Centennial College, Toronto, Canada; [2]University of Toronto, Canada; [3]Centennial College, Toronto, Canada; [4]Sutherland-Chan School, Toronto, Canada; [5]Canadian Memorial Chiropractic College, Toronto, Canada; [6]Coalition of Canadian Herbal Medicine Associations, Canada; [7]Canadian Memorial Chiropractic College, Toronto, Canada; [8]Canadian Memorial Chiropractic College, Toronto, Canada

Aims: CAHC practitioners are increasingly expected to acquire skills in evidence-based practice. Required skills include: digital literacy (computer and web-based skills), research literacy (understanding research language and its application to practice) and research capacity (the ability to design and conduct research studies). Few web-based, sector-specific educational opportunities currently exist. The objective of the project was to evaluate the effect of a ten week asynchronous online course in research literacy for CAHC practitioners on digital and research literacy, cross-sector collaboration and transfer of knowledge to practice. **Methods:** Based on a prospective single group pretest - posttest design, research and digital literacy scores were obtained prior to subjects participating in the online course, again after the course had been completed, and an online survey at six-month follow-up. 34 participants representing 5 CAHC disciplines were originally enrolled in the course, of which 28 participated in the research. Quantitative outcome measures were analyzed descriptively and inferentially using paired t-tests with a one tailed distribution. Descriptive content analysis was conducted on journals and from a focus group. **Results:** Participants reported significant increases in research literacy skills related to finding relevant research (mean increase 28.4%, $p<0.001$), understanding research (38.3%, $p<0.001$) and evaluating research (50.8%, $p<0.001$). In the eight criteria related to digital literacy, significant differences were found in each case ($p<0.001$). Descriptive qualitative content analysis revealed positive self-perceived change in reflective practice; critical thinking skills; profession-specific research advocacy; cross-sector communication and networking; and increased use of research evidence for client/patient education and informed choice. At six month follow-up students continued to feel more confident (n=22, 95.5%, $p<0.001$) in digital and research literacy skills. **Conclusions:** Online learning appears to be an effective strategy for increasing practitioner confidence in digital and research literacy skills, reflective practice, critical thinking, and cross sector communication.

MA9-4

Supporting cancer patients in making safe and informed decisions about complementary and alternative medicine

Balneaves LG[1], Truant TLO[2], Verhoef MJ[3]

[1]School of Nursing, University of British Columbia, Vancouver, Canada; [2]Department of Nursing, British Columbia Cancer Agency, Canada; [3]Department of Community Health Sciences, University of Calgary, Canada

Background: Complementary and alternative medicine (CAM) use has become a common part of cancer patients' experiences. Recent prevalence studies in North America suggest the majority of cancer patients use at least one form of CAM during their disease trajectory. However, despite the growing body of research focused on the decision-making processes of cancer patients regarding complementary and alternative medicine (CAM), there has been little development of interventions that support patients and their significant others in making safe and informed treatment choices related to CAM. **Aims:** The purpose of this paper is to develop recommendations of potential decisional support interventions and educational strategies that will respect patients' decision-making autonomy related to CAM, recognize the social context within which CAM decisions are made, and support patients and their social networks, including health professionals, in making evidence-based CAM treatment decisions. **Methods:** Building on a recently completed systematic review of CAM use within cancer populations (Verhoef, Balneaves, Boon, & Vroegindewey, 2005), recommendations for decisional support interventions will be situated within well-known decision-making theories, including the Ottawa Decision Support Framework, informed by research on the CAM decision-making process in cancer populations, and inspired by the suggestions made by patients themselves regarding the current gaps in supportive care related to CAM in conventional health care settings. In particular, this paper will draw on the past and current research of the authors that has examined the treatment decisions of over 200 Canadian cancer patients using CAM. **Results:** A variety of decisional support interventions and strategies will be presented, including the development of CAM-specific decisional aids for patients and families, the creation of CAM support groups in conventional cancer care centres, and the need for continuing education programs for both conventional and complementary health professionals regarding the use of CAM during cancer. Recommendations that would facilitate more comprehensive and supportive patient-provider communication related to CAM will also be presented. **Conclusions:** With the predominance of CAM use within cancer populations and the growing understanding of the CAM decision-making process, researchers and clinicians must take the next step to develop interventions that will support cancer patients and their social networks in making evidence-based decisions about CAM.

MA9-5

Treat or treatment: A qualitative study conceptualising patients' use of non-medical therapies

Bishop FL[1], Yardley L[2], Lewith GT[3]

[1]Primary Medical Care, [2]School of Psychology, and [3]Primary Medical Care, University of Southampton, UK

Aims: To conceptualise how patients use non-medical therapies and to examine how patients' perspectives relate to existing, expert-led taxonomies. **Methods:** This is a qualitative study with thematic analysis of semi-structured interviews. The study was carried out in two private high-street clinics in the South of England providing a range of non-medical therapies. Purposive sampling was used to recruit 46 people (42 women); they were using aromatherapy massage, herbalism, homeopathy, osteopathy, or reflexology. **Results:** Non-medical therapies appeared to be used in four different ways; as treats, alternative treatments, complementary treatments, and conventional treatments. Treats were portrayed as personal luxuries, not directed at an identified health need, whereas treatments were described as a means of preventing, alleviating or curing specific health problems. There were also systematic differences in the context, anticipated benefits and implications for financial justification when non-medical therapies were viewed and used as alternative, complementary or conventional treatments. There was no simple relationship between patients' ways of using therapies and therapy modality. **Conclusions:** Some people use non-medical therapies as personal luxuries, and not as health care technologies. This way of using non-medical therapies is incongruent with existing expert-led taxonomies. Doctors and researchers need to be aware that patients' views of what constitutes complementary or alternative treatment can differ radically from their own views. They should choose their terminology carefully in order to initiate meaningful dialogue with their patients and research participants. Future research should examine the extent to which the wider population use non-medical therapies as personal luxuries.

MA10-1

Long-term effects of a one-year mind-body medicine program in patients with coronary artery disease: Final results of the randomized controlled SAFE-LIFE trial

Michalsen A, Lehmann N, Paul A, Budde T, Moebus S, Langhorst J, Kerckhoff G, Dobos GJ

Chair of Complementary Medicine, University of Duisburg-Essen; Department of Internal and Integrative Medicine, Kliniken Essen-Mitte, Germany

Aims: The randomized SAFE-LIFE trial tested the effectiveness of an one-year outpatient Integrative Medicine program with focus on Mind-Body Medicine in patients with Coronary Artery Disease (CAD). One-year results showed clinically relevant improvements in cardiac autonomic function, quality of life, need of medication and cardiac symptoms for patients in the intervention group. With the present three-year follow-up we evaluated the long-term effects of the intervention including its impact on coronary artery atherosclerosis **Methods:** 101 patients with medically and interventionally treated CAD were assigned into two groups: 1. Intensive program (IP) group (n=48; 59±8.7 years) with 100 hours lifestyle modification and Mind-body Medicine training over 12 months. 2. Usual care (UC) group (n=53; 59.8±8.6 years) with written information only. Three-year outcomes included blood pressure, heart rate, cardiac symptoms, quality of life and coronary calcification as assessed by coronary electron-beam computed tomography (EBCT). **Results:** Baseline characteristics were comparable. Adherence to proposed lifestyle was still improved after three years in the IP group over UC. Independently of common risk factors, in the IP group a decrease in heart rate ($p<0.01$), systolic blood pressure ($p<0.01$) and diastolic blood pressure ($p<0.05$), a reduced need of medication ($p<0.05$) and a non-significant improvement of quality of life was observed. Both groups showed a comparable age-related progression of the coronary calcium-score. **Conclusion:** A one-year Integrative lifestyle modification program in CAD patients leads to lasting improvements in blood pressure, cardiac autonomic function and need of medication whereas coronary atherosclerosis is not affected. The impact of Integrative lifestyle modification on mortality should be tested in a larger randomized controlled trial.

MA10-2

Prospective randomized three-armed multicentre trial on the influence of a complex naturopathic add-on-therapy during chemotherapy on quality of life in women with breast cancer

Saptania D[1], Reinhard-Hennch B[1], von Hagens C[1], Heym J[1], Adzersen KH[1], Knust U[1], Schneeweiss A[2], Stammer H[2], Abel U[3], van der Haak M[4], Müller A[5], Karcher A[6], Fuxius S[6], Sohn C[2], Strowitzki T[1]

[1]Ambulanz für Naturheilkunde und Integrative Medizin, Abtlg. Gynäkologische Endokrinologie und Fertilitätsstörungen, Universitätsfrauenklinik Heidelberg; [2]Universitätsfrauenklinik Heidelberg; [3]Tumorzentrum Heidelberg/Mannheim, Institut für medizinische Biometrie und Statistik der Universität Heidelberg; [4]Institut für Medizinische Biometrie und Informatik; [5]Geburtshilflich-Gynäkologische Abteilung Krankenhaus Salem Heidelberg; [6]Onkologische Schwerpunktpraxis Heidelberg, Germany

Aims: This trial was carried out to evaluate the influence of a naturopathic add-on-therapy on quality of life, anxiety, depression and laboratory safety parameters during adjuvant, neoadjuvant or palliative chemotherapy in women with breast cancer who frequently use various add-on-therapies. **Patients and methods:** Before starting the chemotherapy 150 women with breast cancer were randomized to 3 groups receiving different add-on interventions during their first 3 cycles of chemotherapy in different units at Heidelberg (University Women's Hospital, Academic Teaching Hospital Salem, oncological practice) from September 2003 until December 2005. Group 1 received an individual consultation about nutrition and physical activity before or at the first day of their chemotherapy and got Na-Selenit 100 g/d, Solidago (goldenrod, 1,680 g/d), Silymarin (milk thistle, 280 mg silibin/d), and Bromelain (pineapple enzyme, 3.000 F.I.P. units/d) as oral medication throughout the first three cycles of the chemotherapy. Group 2 received the same consultation about nutrition and physical activity without medication and group 3 received a leaflet `five-a-day`. Quality of life as primary endpoint was measured with the global health status from the EORTC QLQ-C30 at the first day of the first (baseline) and 3-5 weeks after their third cycle of chemotherapy. Secondary endpoints were other functional and symptom scales of the EORTC QLQ-C30 and BR-23, anxiety and depression measured by the HADS-D (Hospital Anxiety and Depression Scale) and laboratory parameters (hematology, creatinine, SGPT, platelets, Quick(INR), and selenium). **Results:** After the first three cycles of chemotherapy no significant difference in quality of life, anxiety, depression and laboratory parameters could be observed between the three groups. **Conclusions:** An add-on-therapy consisting of a consultation about nutrition and physical activity with and without an oral medication of Na-Selenit (100 g/d), Solidago (1,680 g/d), Silymarin (280 mg silibin/d) and Bromelain (3.000 F.I.P. units/d) during the first three cycles of chemotherapy in breast cancer patients did not have any important clinical benefit on quality of life.

MA10-3

Water drinking cure for alleviating menopausal complaints – a randomised controlled trial

Ortiz M[1], Stange R[1], Woehling H[2], Uehleke B[1]

[1]Department of Natural Medicine, Charité-Universitaetsmedizin Berlin, Campus Benjamin Franklin and Immanuel-Krankenhaus, Berlin, Germany; [2]DABIO contract research organization GmbH, Hoehenkirchen-Siegertsbrunn, Germany

Aims: We investigated the effects of drinking St. Leonhard`s Water in comparison to tap water on menopausal symptoms. St. Leonhard`s Water is a low mineralized water from a natural fontaine in the German prealp region which claims to be helpful against various disorders including menopausal complaints. **Methods:** We conducted a double-blinded, randomised controlled clinical trial in 60 out-patients with a minimum score of 15 on Menopause Rating Scale II (MRS II). Patients were randomised to either drinking 2 liters daily of St. Leonhard`s Water (verum) or 2 liters of tap water (control) using identical looking bottles. Main outcome parameter was change of MRS II after 12 week intervention. The score was evaluated every 3 weeks and at follow up after 9 months. Feasibility and compliance were recorded in a diary. Patients global assessment on change of menopausal symptoms and general well-being was recorded once on a four point scale at the end of intervention. **Results:** 59 out of 60 patients completed the study (age 54.9±5.2, range 46-67). 95% of the patients were postmenopausal evenly distributed to both groups. MRS II for verum decreased significantly by 42.5% (23.2±6.4 to 13.3±6.6; $p<0.01$), as well as for control by 38.3% (24.3±5.3 to 15.0±7.5; $p<0.01$). Mann-Whitney U test showed no statistical difference between groups. Only small changes of the MRS II score (15.1±8.7 for verum, 14.5±7.3 for control) were found in 58 patients at follow up. There was no difference between groups regarding assessment of effects on menopausal complaints. For general well-being the assessment differed slightly in favour of verum. Only 16.6% of verum in contrast to 30% of control assessed no effects of the drinking cure. Compliance and feasibility were good in both groups. The average consumption of water per patient increased from 1.3 liters daily before to 2.7 at the end of study. **Conclusions:** Drinking 2 liters of water daily might have a beneficial effect on menopausal symptoms independent of the type of water. The sustaining effect on menopausal complaints found in the follow up is surprising and may be due to changed drinking habits.

MA10-4

Effectiveness of autologous blood injections (Autohaemotherapy) by acute respiratory tract infections: A randomized, double-blinded, placebo-controlled, multi-centric study

Guendling PW, Hensler S, Schmidt M

Institute for General Practice, Johann Wolfgang Goethe University Hospital, Frankfurt

Background: Autohaemotherapy is a procedure mainly performed in Europe, which is claimed to have therapeutic value for different illnesses, among others acute respiratory tract infections. Until now there have only been a few controlled studies for Autohaemotherapy and there are none for the treatment of acute respiratory tract infections. **Objectives:** To find out whether injections with native autologous blood accelerate the convalescence of patients with acute respiratory tract infections or not. And to find out whether there are any unwanted side effects? **Methods:** The study was carried out in 15 general medical practices in Hesse/Germany with about 160 adult female and male patients aged from 18 to 80 years. Participants with a Jackson-verified acute respiratory tract infection were randomised in two groups and 2 ml blood was taken from everyone. One group of patients immediately received an intragluteal injection of their own blood, the other group was treated in the same way with placebo (0.9% saline solution). This procedure was repeated twice within the following four days. All patients were asked to complete a daily log at the same time, to document the severity of their infection-related symptoms on a 4-point-scale. **Results:** First results suggest that patients treated with Autohaemotherapy recover faster from their infection and that they have no severe side effects. Data will be presented at the conference. **Conclusions:** Autohaemotherapy as a common therapy in German medical practices is an inadequately investigated treatment method. Further investigations are planed.

MA10-5

Effectiveness of cupping therapy in brachialgia paraestetica nocturna: Results of a randomized controlled trial

Michalsen A, Bock S, Lüdtke R, Musial F, Rampp T, Langhorst J, Dobos GJ

Chair of Complementary Medicine, University of Duisburg-Essen; Department of Internal and Integrative Medicine, Kliniken Essen-Mitte, Germany

Aims: Cupping is an established treatment method for regional pain syndromes in various ethnomedical systems worldwide. A pilot study suggested "wet cupping" of a defined connective tissue area (over the Musculus trapezius) to be effective in patients suffering from brachialgia paraesthetica nocturna. We aimed to investigate the effectiveness of this approach by means of a randomized controlled trial. **Methods:** N=52 outpatients (mean age 58.5±8.0y) with manifest chronic brachialgia paraesthetica nocturna and neurologically confirmed carpal tunnel syndrome were enrolled in the study. Patients were randomized into verum or control group and followed up for 7 days. 26 verum patients were treated with a single "wet cupping" treatment in the region of the Musculus trapezius, i.e. the skin was first scarified and then blood was drawn by applying vacuum cupping glasses. 26 control patients were treated with a single local application of a heat pad. Primary outcome measure was mean pre- to post treatment change of brachialgia symptoms including pain, tingling and numbness subscales. Secondary outcomes included neck pain intensity, the functional disability index (DASH-Score) and quality of life (SF-36). **Results:** Symptom severity was reduced from 184.4±61.5 to 73.9±68.0 pts at day 7 in the cupping group and from 201.3±60.6 to 155.1±71.6 pts in the control group (group difference -73.5 pts (95%CI -108.3 to -38.6; $p<0.001$). Highly significant treatment effects were also found for neck pain index (-12.6 pts; 95%CI -18.8 to -6.4; $p<0.001$) and for the functional DASH-Score (-11.1 pts; 95%CI -17.1 to -51; $p<0.001$). The treatment was safe and well tolerated. **Conclusions:** Cupping therapy relieves symptoms in patients with brachialgia paraesthetica nocturna. The potential of cupping for treating brachialgia in the longer term and the related mechanisms remain to be clarified.

MA10-6

Attitudes and preferences of use regarding complementary and alternative medicine (CAM) – a survey among German ambulatory care physicians

Stange R[1], Amhof R[2], Moebus S[3]

[1]Department for Natural Medicine, Charité – Universitaetsmedizin Berlin, Campus Benjamin Franklin and Immanuel-Krankenhaus, Berlin, Germany; [2]Bertelsmann Stiftung, Health Program, Guetersloh, Germany; [3]Institute for Medical Informatics, Biometry and Epidemiology, University Hospital of Essen, University Duisburg-Essen, Germany

Aims: Unconventional medicine - comprised of natural, complementary and alternative medicine - is still gaining popularity among patients and health care providers in western countries. There are many studies investigating patterns of use, e.g. prevalence, expectations, cost and subjective results among general care patients in as well as those with special diseases. Despite this, rather little is known about attitudes and patterns of use among physicians. **Methods:** On the occasion of the yearly "Health care monitor" of the Bertelsmann Stiftung, a representative sample of 516 was drawn from of a basic population of 118,085 German ambulatory care physicians, authorised by the National Association of Statutory Health Insurance Physicians SHI ('Kassenaerztliche Bundesvereinigung') and thus caretaker of appr. 90% of the population – 262 from primary care physicians (general practitioners and general internists, in this case also pediatricians and gynaecologists), 254 from specialists. In November 2005, trained telephone interviewers posed 36 questions in five blocks on personal attitudes and patterns of prescription as well as offers to personally use CAM on patients. **Results:** Out of 512 answers, 51% spoke in favor of CAM (26% 'very much in favor', 25% 'in favor'). Methods most frequently used (combined answers for "I prescribe 'very often', resp. 'at times' ") turned out to be elements of so-called classical natural medicine such as physical therapy (71%), phytomedicine (67%), exercise (63%), nutrition and diets (62%), massage (61%), or relaxation techniques (55%), followed by more typical CAM interventions such as homeopathy (38%), acupuncture (37%) or Traditional Chinese Medicine (18%). Primary care physicians were significantly more inclined to utilise CAM than specialists. This disparity was least for physical therapy, herbal drugs, relaxation techniques, and neural therapy. No striking differences of the usage could be observed with respect to gender or age groups. **Conclusions:** Far more German physicians show acceptance for CAM and offer to personally use it on patients than hitherto believed. Surprisingly, well-known methods traditionally known as 'Natural Medicine' were more frequent than more typical CAM procedures. Further investigations should focus on physicians motivations and differential estimations of results.

MA11-1

Improving homeopathic instruments applying Bayes' theorem

Rutten ALB, Stolper CF, Lugten RF, Barthels RJ

Committee for Methods and Validation, Breda, Netherlands

Aims: Homeopathic clinical experience follows Bayes' theorem, but the repertory is not consistent with this theorem. The Dutch Committee for Methods and Validation uses consensus meetings and prospective research to update the homeopathic repertory according Bayes' rule. **Methods:** 1. Retrospective evaluation since 1997 of 'best' and clear-cut cases. Participants (10–20) apply the nominal group method to evaluate each prescription concerning one medicine. They estimate the prevalence of some symptoms that are known as 'keynotes' in the whole population. We get an indication of the prevalence of the most important symptoms of each medicine from the presented data. 2. Since June 2004, in our prospective study (LR project), 10 experienced homeopathic doctors gather data of all consecutive new patients. Six symptoms are checked in all patients. **Results:** Retrospective analysis of 'best' cases shows that doctors continuously estimate prevalence of symptoms in their practice population and in the populations responding well to specific homeopathic medicines. They implicitly use Bayes' theorem by comparing both populations to estimate chances of cure. Even experienced doctors rarely have more than 3 'best' cases concerning one medicine. Most prescriptions in daily practice are based on symptoms that occur in 1–10% of our population. There is interpersonal variation, caused by chance, especially in daily used symptoms. Gathering results from more doctors should decrease statistical error. Our prospective study shows that the mean values of retrospective estimates were rather accurate, notwithstanding interpersonal variation. Our results did not correspond with the existing repertory in more than 50% of the repertory entries. Applying statistics on our data resulted in new questions like cut-off values for entering new or discarding old entries. **Conclusion:** Repertory entries based on the experience of one expert are liable to statistic error. By gathering of cases of more doctors we can decrease this error. We should apply Bayes' theorem to get reliable results. We need consensus about handling statistical uncertainty.

MA11-2

"She is a human being I can talk to in an ordinary way" – users' experiences with homeopathy

Plunger P

IFF, Palliative Care & Organisational Ethics, University of Klagenfurt, Austria

Aims: The study aims at exploring the views of people with chronic illness and practitioners on homeopathy, and their experiences with homeopathy, taking into account the socio-political, economic and institutional context for homeopathy in Austria. **Methods:** Grounded theory (Strauss 1967) is used, including expert interviews, narrative interviews with users and homeopaths, and a group discussion with homeopaths. Findings from fieldwork are complemented by relevant literature. **Results:** Preliminary findings from interviews with people suffering from chronic illness point out the importance of the doctor-patient relationship: Users emphasise the homeopaths' willingness to take seriously their complaints, their interpretations of illness and the perceived impact of illness on daily life. The concept of trust appears in connection with the users' ability to deal with their illness, the relationship with the homeopath, and the experienced and expected effects of homeopathic treatment. Moreover, trust in the conventional medical system is re-established through the homeopath's referrals to known colleagues. Trust is reproduced and also challenged during the course of treatment, and closely linked to the notions of self-sufficiency, empowerment and self-care. **Conclusions:** Users' expectations and experiences with homeopathic treatment point to key aspects concerning the provision of care for chronically ill people, highlighting the impact of illness on daily life and the fact that this has to be taken into account during the course of treatment. Related to the users' conceptualisations of health and illness, the value of homeopathy is described as ranging from "alternative pharmaceutical treatment" to "some sort of psychotherapy". The case of homeopathy might therefore serve as an example of uncovering users' needs and discussing the potential of integrating complementary and alternative medicine in the provision of care especially for the chronically ill.

MA11-3

The HomBRex basic homeopathy research database in research on the similia principle: A progress report

Van Wijk R[1], Albrecht H[2]

[1]Faculty of Biology, Utrecht University, Utrecht, The Netherlands, [2]Karl and Veronica Carstens Foundation, Essen, Germany

Aims: A search for experimental models that have been used in the study of both proving and therapeutic experiments - ultimately in the research on the homeopathic similia principle. **Methods:** The HomBRex database addressing "Basic Research on Homeopathy" (www.carstens-stiftung.de/hombrex) was used. By the end of 2006 it contained more than 1100 experiments in more than 900 original articles, including 1014 biological studies. **Results:** Biological systems include animal, human, plant, fungi and microbial organisms. Most animal studies (607) were with rat (209) and mouse (171). Most plant studies (171) were with wheat (52). The database highlights whether the experiment was performed on intact organisms or in organs or cells that are for that purpose, isolated and analyzed for changes in structure, function and subcellular composition. The database provides information on 753 experiments utilizing healthy living systems exposed to the substances being tested. These experiments were divided into ideal model proving (497) and prophylactic (256) categories. It also includes 232 therapeutic experiments, in which an effect of a substance was actually tested in a system in a diseased or disturbed state. The database provides information about the disease or disturbance of the system. An overwhelming number of 191 substances were utilized in proving and 112 in therapeutic experiments. Those include high and low dilutions and potencies. **Conclusion:** In general, basic research in homeopathy does not directly address the simile principle. It is concluded that from the overwhelming variety in organisms, diseased states, and substances, only a limited number of biological systems and states might be sufficiently used in therapeutic as well as in proving studies to allow the question, which model organisms have sufficient data to study the similia principle.

MA11-4

Homeopathic pathogenetic trials produce more specific than non-specific symptoms: Results from two double-blind placebo controlled pathogenetic trials

Walach H, Möllinger H, Sherr J, Schneider R

University of Northampton, School of Social Sciences & Samueli Institute, European Office

Aims: To determine whether symptoms reported by healthy volunteers produced by homeopathic remedies were significantly different for homeopathic remedies from placebos. **Methods:** We conducted two parallel, blinded and randomised homeopathic experimental, i.e. pathogenetic trials conducted at two different sites. Substances potentised to 30C were selected blindly and randomly from a pre-determined list of 20 potential remedies by an independent party. Study 1 ($n=17$) employed a two-armed design, testing ozone against placebo. Study 2 ($n=36$) employed a three-armed design, testing ozone and iridium against placebo. Volunteers were contacted on a daily basis by supervisors and potential symptoms were established into a diary. An independent specialist for homeopathic materia medica determined blindly for each reported symptom, whether it was a symptom specific for the remedy tested or not. This yielded the target variable: number of remedy specific symptoms per group. **Results:** We found significantly more remedy specific symptoms in provers taking ozone or iridium than in provers taking placebo in the three-armed trial ($p=0.0015$; Kruskal Wallis) and in both trials pooled for ozone and placebo ($p=0.011$; Mann-Whitney). **Conclusion:** Homeopathic remedies produce more symptoms typical for a remedy than non-typical symptoms. The results furthermore suggest a somewhat non-classical pattern because symptoms of one remedy appear to be mimicked in a preceding baseline phase or in the other trial arm. This is indicative of entanglement in homeopathic systems for which previously indications have been found.

MA11-5

Homeopathy as an adjuvant to chemotherapy improves clinical outcome in relapsed pulmonary tuberculosis

Sharma N, Sharma RG, Sharma S, Chand K

University of Rajasthan, Jaipur, India

Aim: To investigate the efficacy of homeopathy as complementary medicine in relapse pulmonary tuberculosis. **Methods:** In a randomized placebo control study, 47 patients with relapse pulmonary tuberculosis were given homeopathy (24) or placebo (23) for 6 months in addition to conventional chemotherapy. Primary outcomes were sputum conversion, weight gain and haematological assessment (Erythrocytic sedimentation rate and hemoglobin). Secondary outcome measures were symptoms of cough, night sweat, chest pain, breathlessness, haemoptysis, fever and quality of life. Measurements were carried out before and after 2 and 6 months of anti- tuberculosis treatment. Patients were also followed for 3 months after anti-tuberculosis treatment. **Results:** Compared with placebo group the homeopathy group showed significant improvement defined as increased body weight (p<0.001), higher sputum conversion rate (87.5%) and faster reduction of symptoms (p<0.001). There was a significant improvement in homeopathy group in all domains of quality of life such as body pain, energy, general health, mental health, physical function, social function, role limitation physical and role limitation emotional compared to placebo. At follow up 12.5% patients on homeopathy were remained sputum positive compared to 52.2% on placebo. **Conclusion:** Homeopathy as a supplement to anti-tuberculosis chemotherapy given to relapsed pulmonary tuberculosis patients may represent a valuable and cost effective treatment strategy that might shorten the duration of conventional treatment by enhancing mycobacterial host defense. Enhanced sputum conversion and reduced cough may reduce the transmission of smear positive tuberculosis.

MA11-6

Effects of homeopathic herbal preparations on human prostate cancer growth in vivo

Amri H[1], MacLaughlin B[1], Anderson N[1], Ives J[2], Jonas W[2]

[1]Department of Physiology and Biophysics, Georgetown University Medical Center, Washington, USA; [2]Samueli Institute for Information Biology, Alexandria, USA

Background: Worldwide prostate cancer related deaths have been estimated at 204,000/year. Conventional medicine relies on prostate specific antigen measurements and biopsies to diagnose the disease and offers a disease management plan, based on patient age and comorbidity. In integrative and complementary medicine, homeopaths use herbals to treat prostate problems ranging from benign prostatic hyperplasia to cancer. In this study wc aim to assess the antiproliferative effects of Sabal serrulata (Ss), Thuja occidentalis (Toc), and Conium maculatum (Cm) on nude mice xenografts of PC-3 human prostate cancer cells and decipher the molecular mechanism(s) of action. **Methods:** Male nude mice were inoculated with either PC-3 human prostate or MDA-MB-231 human breast cancer cells as control. The animals were divided into several experimental groups (n=10) to receive daily gavage treatment of either Ss (200CH) only, or a multitreatment (MT) of Toc (1000CK), Cm (1000CK), Ss (200CH), and carcinosin (1000CK) on a weekly schedule. Untreated animals and treated with successed water (200CH) were included as controls. The treatment was carried out for 5 weeks followed by five observation weeks. The tumor size was measured and the animal weights recorded. Animals underwent MRI scanning to visualize the tumors. After completion of the experiment, the tumors, serum, plasma, and metastatic lesions were collected. Proliferating cell nuclear antigen (PCNA) and apoptosis using TUNEL staining are being performed. **Results:** The tumor incidence rate in the untreated group was at 100%, remained at 75% for the Ssl, 94% for the MT, and 83% for the successed water. When compared to the untreated control group, tumor growth in the Ss only group decreased to 42% (p=0.012) but was marginally significant when Ss was administered bi-weekly as part of the MT (p=0.07). No effect was observed on breast cancer tumor growth. MRI results confirmed the tumor measurements. The PCNA staining showed about 30% decrease in cell proliferation in the Ss only group as compared to both untreated and successed water controls. **Conclusion:** Our study demonstrates a biologic response to homeopathic treatment which was significantly stronger to Ss and specific to human prostate cancer. The next steps for this study would be the elucidation of the antitumorigenic mechanisms using functional genomics and proteomics.

MA12-1

Integrative medicine – medicine of the future?

Dobos GJ

Chair of Complementary Medicine, University of Duisburg-Essen; Department of Internal and Integrative Medicine, Kliniken Essen-Mitte, Germany

An analysis of the prevalent illnesses in the western world shows a significant shift during the past few decades. Due to the enormous progress in modern medicine, acute infectious diseases have become less threatening; the number of deaths they cause is decreasing steadily whereas chronic diseases are developing into a new scourge in the Western culture. Most of the over 65-year-olds are suffering from chronic illnesses, which causes an explosion in medical care cost. In Germany about 80% of the expenses of the health system are spent on chronically ill patients. This situation is not merely a financial problem, but a new challenge for physicians since a large percentage of patients suffering from chronic diseases benefits from conventional therapies only to a limited degree. Moreover, long-term medication rarely leads to a complete cure of the illness treated and chronically ill patients are often exposed to long-term polymedication that causes interactions between the prescribed substances which scientifically still are not fully known and understood. Official figures show that in the U.S. over 100,000 patients die annually because of side effects of their medication. Integrative Medicine is a new approach in the treatment of common chronic, as well as acute illnesses. It employs proven methods and procedures developed within the therapeutic systems of Complementary Medicine (Complementary and Alternative Medicine or CAM) and of Mind/Body Medicine, which helps patients to develop skills in improving the self-healing capacity of the body and in coping with illnesses through behavioural methods. Metaphorically the term "Integrative Medicine" can be understood as a multilingualism. An integrative physician uses several different "languages" to understand and to treat a patient and his disease/s. Decisions about the most appropriate methods are based on both the relevant scientific evidence (external evidence) as well as on the physician's own experience (internal evidence). According to our experience Integrative Medicine is effective, cost effective and side-effects of medication in patients with chronic illnesses are reduced. Integrative Medicine may therefore serve as a model for the future.

MA12-2

The profiles of GP-only users, CAM practitioner-only users and patients who use both: A comparative total population based study (HUNT 2)

Steinsbekk A[1], Adams J[2], Sibbritt D[3], Jacobsen G[1], Johnsen R[1]

[1]Norwegian University of Science and Technology (NTNU), Department of Public Health and General Practice, Trondheim, Norway; [2]School of Population Health, University of Queensland, Australia; [3]Centre for Clinical Epidemiology and Biostatistics, School of Medicine and Public Health, Faculty of Health, University of Newcastle, Australia

Objective: To compare the profiles of people visiting only a general practitioner (GP), those visiting only a practitioner of complementary and alternative medicine (CAM) and those visiting both (GP&CAM). **Methods:** Design: A comparative total population health survey in central Norway (HUNT 2). Subjects: 54,448 persons 20 years of age and over who answered questions about their use of health services during the previous 12 months. Variables: Sociodemographic characteristics, self perceived health, subjective health complaints, and a variety of common diseases**. Results:** 34 854 (64.0%) of those who answered the health service use question had visited only a GP, 837 (1.5%) only a CAM practitioner and 4563 (8.4%) both during the last 12 months. The likelihood of being a CAM-only user as compared to a GP-only user was significantly increased (p<0.005) if the participant was male; aged between 30 and 69; and without cardiovascular disease. The likelihood of being a GP&CAM user compared to GP-only user was significantly increased (p<0.005) for those being female; aged between 30 and 59; had higher education level; was a non-smokers; had lower perceived global health; had limiting chronic complaint; had experienced a health complaint during the last 12 months; had musculoskeletal disease; had psychiatric complaint; and had hay fever. **Conclusion:** There were few CAM-only users and they differ from GP-only users by being male, aged 30-69 and without cardiovascular disease. Users of both GP&CAM were less healthy with more complaints and poorer self reported health than GP and CAM-only users.

MA12-3

Issues in interface between Western medicine and traditional Korean medicine in Korea: What are health policy options for a new integrative health system?

Han D, Yoon TH, Choi B, Chung E, Kim Y

Hanynag University, College of Medicine and Institute of Health Care Management, Seoul, Korea; National Traditional Korean Medicine Research and Development Center

Background and aims: As a global issue, many countries are facing the demand for reshaping health care systems to cope with rapid changes in health care sector. The recent growth of oriental medicine and complementary and alternative medicine (CAM) in the many countries is, to a large extent, due to the growth of the number of oriental medical doctors and physicians who have taken up alternative therapies alongside conventional medicine. To cope with the changing environments, many countries consider developing integrative health care which is now used widely in health care sector. In both biomedical and CAM sectors (including oriental medicine), attention appears to have shifted away from separating therapeutic modalities into categories such as biomedical or CAM, towards a focus on merging diverse modalities into a "new" integrative health system. In Korea, one of peculiar characteristics of health care system is that as health care provider, traditional Korean medicine and western medicine coexist since 19th century. Recently, the government of Korea has given many efforts to enhance the role and function of traditional Korean medicine in public health care sector. However, the strategies and measures for integrative health care settings combining traditional Korean medicine and western medicine on health sector have not been developed yet. The research question of this study is: In Korea, what are the trends and problems in interface of traditional Korean medical sector and Western medical sector; what are the causes of or associated factors to the problems; how to cope with the problems and how to resolve the causes?; what are the health policy directions and its strategies that the government should take to cope with the future demand and the burden on health care sector? **Methods:** In order to do this, this study explores the current situations and issues on the interface between traditional Korean medicine and (western) medicine in various ways using contents analysis of existing data and documents related to traditional Korean medicine and health policy. **Results and Conclusion:** We discussed stakeholders' views on the interface in the health care sector. Then, health policy options have to shift away from separating therapeutic modalities into categories such as "traditional Korean medicine" or 'western medicine", towards a focus on merging diverse modalities into a "new" integrative health system.

MA12-4

Bridge building and integrative treatment approaches in Denmark and Norway – research designs, results and lessons learned

Nyborg L, Launsø L

NAFKAM, University of Tromsø, Norway

A trend moving towards developing bridge building and integrative treatment is taken place internationally including cooperation between conventional and alternative practitioners in hospital settings and between hospitals and private sectors. However, systematic research-based evaluations of integrative treatment efforts have yet to be carried out. No blueprint exists on how to develop bridge-building processes in which cooperation is initiated and developed between conventional and alternative practitioners within the health care system. Results from two empirical studies undertaken in Denmark and Norway on bridge building and integrative treatment will be presented. In cooperation with researchers the Danish Multiple Sclerosis Society (a patient-association) has initiated a research project on bridge building and integrative treatment. A team has been developed including ten practitioners, one medical doctor (neurologist), one occupational therapist, one physical therapist, one psychologist, one nurse and one acupuncturist, one nutritional therapist, one classical homeopath, one cranio-sacral therapist, and one reflexologist. The research questions are: 1) What can the practitioners learn from participating in a bridge-building project and from developing an integrative treatment approach to persons with MS (PwMS)? 2) How do the practitioners assess practitioner-researcher seminars as a tool for developing bridge building and integrative treatment approach to PwMS? The experiences from the Danish research project have been used in a Norwegian context where the National Research Centre on Complementary and Alternative Medicine (NAFKAM), University of Tromsø, Norway has initiated a research project on hospital departments in Norway initiating social experiments on integrative treatment. The aim of the first phase of this project is to obtain knowledge of the content of the ongoing activities in hospitals and the healthcare professionals' motivations, knowledge, and attitudes to integrative treatment. Also the actors' experiences and the facilitating and prohibiting factors in the establishment of these innovative treatment approaches are investigated. Research designs and results from the two projects will be outlined followed by lessons learned from undertaken these kinds of research projects.

MA12-5

Towards a model for integrative medicine in Swedish primary care

Sundberg T[1], Halpin J[2], Warenmark A[3], Falkenberg T[1]

[1]Center for Studies of Complementary Medicine, Department of Neurobiology, Care Sciences and Society, Division of Nursing, Karolinska Institutet, Sweden; [2]Axelsons Gymnastiska Institut, Stockholm, Sweden, and Center för Energimedicin, Stockholm, Sweden; [3]Rågsveds Husläkare, Bandhagen, Sweden

Aims: Collaboration between providers of conventional care and complementary therapies (CTs) has gained in popularity but there is a lack of conceptualized models for delivering such care, i.e. integrative medicine (IM). The overall aim of the current research has been to develop and implement an IM model adapted to Swedish primary care (completed) and evaluate it through a randomised clinical trial (completed, analysis pending). This abstract reports some key findings relevant to the development and implementation of the proposed IM model. **Methods:** Investigative procedures involved research group and key informant meetings with multiple stakeholders, ie general practitioners, CT providers, medical specialists, primary care administrators and county council representatives. Data collection included meeting notes which were feedbacked within the research group and used as ongoing working documents. Data analysis was made by immersion/crystallization and research group consensus. Results were categorized within a public health systems framework of structures, processes and outcomes. **Results:** Structures: CT centers were established at Stockholm county council and Karolinska Institutet along with CT utilization prevalence research and CT courses for medical students and health care providers. Processes: Interaction between conventional and CT providers resulted in a research group which developed and implemented an IM model adapted to Swedish primary care. Outcomes: The developed IM model aims for a patient centered interdisciplinary non-hierarchical mix of conventional and complementary medical solutions to individual case management of low back and neck pain. The IM model adhere to standard clinical practice with active partnership between a gate keeping general practitioner collaborating with a team of CT providers in a consensus case conference model of care. CTs with an emerging evidence base included in the IM model were Swedish massage therapy, manual therapy (naprapathy), shiatsu, acupuncture and qigong. **Conclusions:** The development of the proposed IM model was facilitated by the county council CT center recommending dialogue on IM, and the academic CT center and course providing the basis for research and development. The proposed IM model is currently evaluated in a pragmatic randomised controlled trial to explore its clinical effectiveness.

PG1-01

Chronoprotective effects of pomegranate juice on iodoacetate-induced osteoarthritis on tibiofemoral joint of mice

Hadipour-Jahromy M, Safavi M, Shirin-Kalam M, Nazer N, Shirzadian F

Islamic Azad University, Teheran, Iran

Aims: To study the effectiveness of Pomegranate juice (PJ) on osteoarthritis (OA), we used mono-iodoacetate (MIA), an inhibitor of glycolysis, in tibiofemoral joint of mice that promotes loss of articular cartilage similar to that noted in human OA. Pomegranate juice (PJ) is increasing in popularity because of its high antioxidant content, already known to help prevent heart disease. The fruit is native to the area between Iran and northern India. Pomegranate fruit extract (PFE) was recently shown to exert anti-inflammatory effects in different disease models and protect chondrocytes in vitro. However, no histopathological studies have been undertaken in vivo to investigate whether PJ protect articular cartilage. **Methods:** We describe the histopathology in the subchondral bone and cartilage of mice knee joints treated with a single intra-articular injection of MIA (1 mg) and sacrificed at 1, 14 and 28 days post injection. Then, the beneficial effect of PJ (without seeds) was studied in different groups, orally; Group 1: administration of PJ (4ml/kg), Group 2: administration of PJ (20 ml/kg). Histopathological changes in knee joints were studied after two and four weeks. **Results:** Histologically, the early OA were characterized by areas of chondrocytes degeneration/necrosis sometimes involving the entire thickness of the articular cartilage in the tibial plateaus and femoral condyles. Changes to the subchondral bone and proteoglycane contents, were observed and also, there was focal fragmentation and collapse of bony trabeculae with fibrosis and necrosis. Synovial cell proliferation was noted. Interestingly, administration of PJ in different groups of mice prevented the negative effects of iodoacetate, both dose and time dependently. Chondrocytes damages were significantly prevented and proteoglycanes were less affected, especially in groups receiving high amount of PJ and no cell proliferation and inflammatory cell were detected in synovial. **Conclusions:** Fast and progressive damage to articular cartilage is induced by single intra-articular injection of MIA, which mimic exactly human OA. In this study, the effectiveness of PJ in improvement of histopathological damages is emphasized and its chondroprotective effect in vivo is highlighted.

PG1-02

Anti-inflammatory activity of flower tops of Gentiana Kurroo Royale extract

Latif A, Khan TF, Afaq SH

Department of Ilmul Advia, A.K. Tibbiya College, Faculty of Unani Medicine, Aligarh Muslim University, India

Background: *Gentiana Kurroo* Royale (GK) flower tops (Gule-Ghafis) has been traditionally used for the treatment of inflammation, pain, fever and hepatitis in Unani System of Medicine. The plant was sold in Eastern countries under the name Gul-Ghafis which is *Gentiana daliurica* Fisch. But sample obtained from the major cities of India were found and identified as flower tops of *Gentiana Kurroo* Roy ale. However this work was aimed at the scientific validation of ethanopharmacological claim about the anti-inflammatory property of *Gentiana Kurroo* Royal flower tops extract. **Methods:** Air-dried flower tops of GK were blended to a fine powder extracted with 50% ethanol. The phytochemical screening, quantitative estimation (%) TLC and anti-inflammatory screening were investigated. The study was carried out on Wistar rats of either sex. Animals were divided into three groups of six each. Rat paw edema induced by Carrageenan 0.1 ml of 1% carrageenan in 0.9% NaCl was administered into planter surface of right hind paw. The experimental groups-I was fed with extract in the dose of 1000 mg/ kg body weight, the animal in group-II served as control group and administered with 20 ml/ kg distilled water while standard drug Diclofenac sodium was given to group-III in the dose of 5 mg/ kg orally an hour prior to administration of carrageenan. After injection animals were observed and readings were obtained for each rat at 60, 120, 180, 240 and 300 minutes with the aid of Plethysmometer. The percentage of inhibition for each rats were calculated by the formula of New Bould (1963). **Results:** The phytochemical screening revealed the presence of alkaloids, flavonoids, glycosides, free phenols, sterols/ terpens. Percentage estimated as alkaloid 0.33±0.02, phenols 2.9±0.07, sterols/ terpens 1.35±0.01, flavonoid 0.34±0.24 were found. Thin layer chromatography of flavonoid fraction showed Robinetin-0, Luteolin, Apigenin, Kaempferol and Kaempferid. The effect of extract of flower tops of GK showed a maximum anti-inflammatory effect about 68.58% ($p<0.01$) at 180 min. while the anti-inflammatory effect of Diclofenac sodium reached a maximum 70.58% ($p<0.01$) at 180 min. **Conclusions:** The results indicate that the flower tops of GK posses anti-inflammatory activity against inflammation induced by carrageen an in acute phase. Thus, this study strongly indicates the non-steroidal anti-inflammatory activity. They may act by the inhibition of production of prostaglandins, other than this the presence of flavonoids may account for its anti-inflammatory pharmacological activity. This pharmacological study is validating the claims of ancient Unani Physicians regarding the anti inflammatory property of the *Gentiana Kurroo* Royale flower tops.

PG1-03

Preclinical analyses of Essiac®, a commonly used herbal anti-cancer formula

Seely D[1,2], Kennedy DA[1], Myers SP[3], Cheras PA[3], Lin D[3], Li R[3], Cattley T[3], Brent PP[3], Leonard BJ[4]

[1]Department of Research and Clinical Epidemiology, The Canadian College of Naturopathic Medicine, Toronto, Canada; [2]Institute of Medical Science, University of Toronto, Canada; [3]Australian Centre for Complementary Medicine, Southern Cross University, Lismore NSW, Australia; [4]Faculty of Medicine, University of Toronto, Canada

Objective: Essiac® is an herbal compound that has been in common use with cancer patients in North America for over 80 years. Despite widespread use, there is very limited evidence to support or oppose the use of this herbal formula. We aimed to address the lack of evidence with a series of in vitro and in vivo experiments to assess for physiological activity and potential for harm. **Methods** (in vitro): The activity of Essiac® was quantified with respect to antioxidant activity, inhibition of platelet aggregation, anti-microbial activity, inhibition of the arachidonic acid pathway, cell-based immunomodulation, neoplastic cell specific cytotoxicity, fibrinolytic activity, and inhibition of cytochrome P450 enzymes. **Results** (in vitro): Essiac® exhibited significant antioxidant activity using the ABTS assay. Essiac® at also exhibited significant immunomodulatory effects, specifically through stimulation of granulocyte phagocytosis (28.24±0.26%), increases in CD8+ cell activation (>5-fold), and via moderate inhibition of COX-1 (18±1%), COX-2 (24±0.5%), 5-lipoxygenase (16±1%), and phospholipase A2 enzyme activity (12±0.5%). Essiac® also exhibited significant cell specific cytotoxicity towards ovarian epithelial carcinoma cells (A2780) and prostate adenocarcinoma cells (PC3). A 20-fold dilution of Essiac® also inhibited several cytochrome P450 enzymes, most notably CYP1A2 (37%) and CYP2C19 (24%). Essiac® demonstrated dose-dependent inhibition of clot fibrinolysis, with significant inhibition exhibited at 1:40 dilution. Essiac® demonstrated no changes in platelet aggregation nor any anti-microbial activity. **Methods** (in vivo): Wistar rats were used to test for protection against ethanol induced gastric ulceration and carbon tetrachloride induced hepatic injury. Assays to assess post-glucose-load serum glucose, and cellular and humoral immune modulation were conducted on ICR and BALB/C mice respectively. **Results** (in vivo): Essiac® demonstrated a modest gastric protective effect via reduction of ethanol induced gastric ulceration. Essiac® did not demonstrate significant hepatoprotective, hypoglycaemic, or immunomodulatory properties. **Conclusions:** The in vivo study is significant as it represents the first published investigation of Essiac® in an animal model. Some evidence of protection against gastric ulceration was found and no evidence of harm was demonstrable. The in vitro analysis of Essiac®, the first comprehensive preclinical investigation of its potential anti-cancer role, indicated significant antioxidant and immunomodulatory properties, as well as neoplastic cell specific cytotoxicity consistent with its historically ascribed properties. Evidence of cytochrome P450 and fibrinolysis inhibition was observed.

PG1-04

Gypenoside XLIX from Gynostemma pentaphyllum, modulates pro-atherosclerotic mediators via a PPAR-alpha-dependent pathway

Roufogalis BD, Huang TH-W, Tran VH, Li Q, Li Y

Herbal Medicines Research and Education Centre, Faculty of Pharmacy, University of Sydney, NSW, Australia

Atherosclerosis is an inflammatory process triggered by the presence of lipids in the vascular wall and encompasses a complex interaction between inflammatory cells, vascular elements and lipoproteins through the expression of several adhesion molecules and cytokines, including tissue factor (TF) and vascular cell adhesion molecule 1 (VCAM-1). Activation of the nuclear receptor peroxisome proliferator-activated receptor (PPAR)-alpha has been demonstrated to modulate many aspects of lipoprotein metabolism and inflammation in vitro as well as in animal and human studies. PPAR-alpha mediates many anti-inflammatory and anti-atherogenic effects. Gynostemma pentaphyllum (GP) has been clinically shown to reduce total cholesterol, triglyceride and low density lipoprotein levels and increase high density lipoprotein, and is widely used in the treatment of various inflammatory and cardiovascular diseases, including atherosclerosis. Recently, we demonstrated that GP extract (gypenosides) and Gypenoside (Gyp)-XLIX, a dammarane-type glycoside, are potent PPAR-alpha activators. In this study the effect of Gyp-XLIX has been investigated against a number of pro-atherosclerotic mediators. Gyp-XLIX (0–300 micromolar) concentration-dependently inhibited tissue factor (TF) promoter activity after induction by the inflammatory stimulus lipopolysaccharide (LPS) in human monocytic THP-1 cells transfected with promoter reporter constructs pTF-LUC. Furthermore, Gyp-XLIX inhibited LPS-induced overexpression of TF mRNA and protein in THP-1 monocyte cells. On the other hand, Gyp-XLIX inhibited VCAM-1 promoter activity after induction by cytokine tumor necrosis factor (TNF)-alpha in human umbilical vein endothelial cells (HUVECs) transfected with promoter reporter construct pVCAM-1-LUC. Moreover, Gyp-XLIX inhibited TNF-alpha-induced VCAM-1 mRNA and protein overexpression in HUVECs. We show that the activities of Gyp-XLIX are similar to those of Wy-14643, a potent synthetic PPAR-alpha activator. The activities of both Gyp-XLIX and Wy-14643 were completely abolished by a selective blocker of PPAR-alpha, MK-886. Thus, our findings suggest that Gyp-XLIX modulates pro-atherosclerotic mediators via a PPAR-alpha-dependent pathway. These data provide new insight into the rational basis of the use of the traditional Chinese herbal medicine Gynostemma pentaphyllum in the treatment of atherosclerosis, as well as other inflammatory and cardiovascular diseases.

PG1-05

An isopropanolic extract of black cohosh (iCR) that induces apoptosis and decreases growth and invasiveness of human breast cancer cells as an option for the treatment of women with a history of breast cancer

Hostanska K[1], Nisslein T[2], Freudenstein J[2], Reichling J[3], Saller R[1]

[1]Institute for Complementary Medicine, University Hospital Zurich, Switzerland; [2]Schaper & Brümmer GmbH & Co.KG, Salzgitter, Germany; [3]Institute of Pharmacy and Molecular Biotechnology, University of Heidelberg, Germany

Background: Breast cancer is the most common malignancy affecting women. Hormone replacement therapy is contraindicated in women with breast cancer. Extracts from rhizomes of black cohosh *Actaea syn. Cimicifuga racemosa* (CR), have gained acceptance as a natural alternative for the treatment and prevention of menopausal disorders. **Materials and Methods:** Isopropanolic-aqueous extract iCR (B.Nr.231050; 77 mg/ml dry residue), fractions of triterpene glycosides (TTG; 27mg/ml) and cinnamic acid esters (CAE; 3.7 mg/ml) were provided by Schaper & Brümmer GmbH & Co KG (Salzgitter, Germany). Estrogen receptor-positive (ER^+) MCF-7 and estrogen receptor-negative (ER^-) MDA MB 231 human breast adenocarcinoma cells were from ATCC (Rockville, USA). Cell growth inhibition and apoptosis induction were investigated after 72h incubation using WST-1 and/or crystal violet and annexin V adhesion by flow cytometry and/or morphological assessment of apoptosis. M30-Apoptosense ELISA (PEVIVA, Alexis Corp., Basel) was used for the measurement of the M30 neoepitope which is associated with caspase-activation. The effect of test substances upon the invasive potential of MDA-MB231 cells was studied in BD Biocoat Matrigel™ (BD, Bedford, USA) invasion chambers over a period of 24h. **Results:** iCR significantly inhibited breast cancer cell proliferation. The effects were clearly dose-dependent with a 50 % growth inhibitory concentration (IC_{50}) of 54.1±11.4 µg/ml in MCF-7 cells and of 29.5±3.0 µg/ml in MDA-MB231 cells, respectively. Both, TTG and CAE fractions inhibited growth of MCF-7 cells, the IC_{50} being 59.3 µg/ml and 26.1 µg/ml. Further, the mode of cell death was identified as apoptosis by microscopic inspection and confirmed by light scatter characteristics and by detection of Annexin V adherence to phosphatidylserine by flow cytometry. In addition, the involvement of activated caspases was demonstrated by the cleavage of cytokeratin 18 as detected with M30 antibody. Increases in the level of M30-antigen of about 4-fold and 2-fold over untreated controls were observed in iCR-treated MCF-7 and MDA-MB231 cells. The invasive capacity of MDA-MB231 cells was suppressed by 51.8% at 77.4 µg/ml of iCR, an extract concentration where 89% of cells were viable. At a dose of 5 µg/ml, TTG and CAE reduced cell invasion by 34% and 25.5%, respectively. **Conclusion:** These results indicate that iCR extract exerts no proliferative activity, but kills the ER^+ MCF-7 as well as ER^- MDA-MB231 cells by activation of caspases and induction of apoptosis.TTG and CAE compounds significantly contribute to its apoptotic effect. Antiinvasive activity together with the antiproliferative and apoptosis-inducing effect of iCR suggest its use as a secure agent in postmenopausal hormone replacement therapy with additional chemopreventive activity.

PG1-06

Efficacy of Fenugreek Galactomannan formulations in the obesity management

Ngondi JL, Oben J

Department of Biochemistry, Faculty of Science, University of Yaounde I, Cameroon

Objective: Fenugreek (Trigonella foenum-graecum) has a long history of medical uses in Ayurvedic and Chinese medicine, and has been used for numerous indications. Preliminary animal and human trials suggest possible hypoglycemic and antihyperlipidemic properties of oral fenugreek seed powder. This study investigated the effect of Fenugreek galactomannan formulations on weight loss and the composition of biochemical parameters related to weight loss. **Research Design and Methods:** We conducted a seven week double blind placebo trial where 25 obese subjects treated conventionally by a low fat diet were randomly assigned to take either fenugreek formulations in capsules or placebo. To achieve moderate caloric restriction (1800–2000 Kcal/day) individual dietary counselling was also done. The diet was controlled by a seven days food diary. The drug and the placebo capsules were indistinguishable both for the patient and the physician. There were five types of capsules named Fenugreek (F), Fenugreek + phaseolamine (F+P), Fenugreek + Commiphora mukul + ayurverdic fruit mix (F+G+A), Commiphora mukul + ayurverdic fruit mix (G+A) and placebo. **Results:** Subjects who received placebo capsules showed a mean decrease in body weight of 1.32±0.41% ($p<0.02$) after two weeks of treatment where as those on fenugreek formulations showed a decrease in weight comprised between 1.6±0.4% ($p<0.001$) and 2.82±1.05% ($p<0.001$). For active drugs groups weight loss was maintained through out the end of the experimental period and the mean decrease in body weight comprised between 4.83±1.07% and 5.87±0.71% was significantly different from that of placebo group 2.2% ±1.05% ($p<0.05$). An improvement in blood pressure was observed with fenugreek formulations in capsules. The primary blood pressure end point (systolic blood pressure) decreased significantly with G+A (12.42±4.2 mmHg; $p<0.02$), Fenugreek (13±6.1 mmHg ($p<0.05$) and the diastolic blood pressure with F (8.53 ±4.2 mmHg; $p<0.05$), F+P (13.15±6.16 mmHg; $p<0.05$), F+G+A (5.1±2.13 mmHg; $p<0.05$). There were significant changes in total cholesterol, LDL cholesterol, HDL cholesterol, and triglycerides when the active formulations in capsules were compared with the placebo. **Conclusion:** Fenugreek formulations aresafe and effective in weight reduction. They may help, retard, prevent or treat obesity.

PG1-07

Cholesterol reduction through psyllium husks – is there a compliance problem because of adverse gastrointestinal effects?

Uehleke B, Ortiz M, Stange R

Department of Natural Medicine, Charite University Medicine Berlin, Germany

Aims: The use of psyllium husks (Plantaginis ovatae testa) in hypercholesterolemia is rather rare in comparison to their use as a laxative. This might be due to either insufficient effects or to gastrointestinal adverse effects such as meteorism and diarrhea. **Methods:** We conducted an observational study in 60 out-patients with both indications – hypercholesterolemia and constipation – with emphasis on gastrointestinal symptoms. The main outcome parameters were total cholesterol and LDL after 3 weeks intake of 3.5 g psyllium husks t.i.d. without a change in diet. For the documentation of gastrointestinal symptoms before and after therapy we used part 1 of the validated Nepean Dyspepsia Index (Talley 1999) addressing intensity, frequency, and impact of 15 dyspeptic symptoms of the upper abdominal region during the last two weeks. In an analogous manner we added 10 questions about symptoms of irritable bowel. Patients recorded gastrointestinal symptoms in a diary. Compliance and motivation were also evaluated. **Results:** 54 out of 62 patients finished the study showing a significant ($p<0.001$) reduction from 252 to 239 mg/dl for total cholesterol and from 174 to 162 mg /dl for LDL. HDL and triacylglycerol remained unchanged. The total gastrointestinal symptoms score was lower after 3 weeks of therapy (27) than before (24). Diaries showed various gastrointestinal symptoms in the first week of treatment decreasing during week 2 and week 3. A small increase of defecation frequency from week 1 to week 3 was observed. There were 26 gastrointestinal adverse drug reactions during the first week, which were relieved in the further course. 80 % of patients would consider long-term treatment with this natural product. **Conclusions:** We confirmed the known cholesterol lowering effects of psyllium husks. Long-term effects on cholesterol are expected to be higher than those observed in our study after 3 weeks. Patients with a sensitive gastrointestinal system or functional gastrointestinal disorders show initial but transient adverse gastrointestinal effects. Patients with functional disorders, e.g. constipation, can expect a positive influence on their symptoms, e.g. stool frequency and consistency. It is, however, important that patients are well informed about the transient nature of possible adverse gastrointestinal effects, which might be reduced by a gradual increase of the dosage.

PG1-08

Bromelain as an adjunctive treatment for moderate-to-severe osteoarthritis of the knee: A randomized placebo-controlled pilot study

Brien S, Lewith G, Walker AF, Middleton R, Prescott P, Bundy R

University of Southampton, UK

Background: Osteoarthritis (OA) of the knee is the most prevalent joint disorder worldwide. Bromelain, an extract from the pineapple plant, has purported anti-inflammatory and analgesic properties. Previous uncontrolled studies suggest it may provide safe and effective treatment for OA knee. **Aim:** To assess the specific efficacy of Bromelain as an adjunctive treatment for osteoarthritis of the knee. **Methods:** Randomised, placebo controlled trial. 47 subjects with a confirmed diagnosis of moderate to severe OA knee were entered into this double-blind, randomized placebo-controlled study. Subjects were randomised and received twelve weeks of treatment intervention (Bromelain 800 mg/d or placebo) with a four-week follow-up period. Knee (pain, stiffness and function) and quality of life symptoms were reported monthly within WOMAC and SF-36. Adverse events were recorded. The primary outcome measure was the change in total WOMAC score from baseline to the end of treatment at week 12. Longitudinal equation modelling was used to evaluate outcome. **Results:** 31 patients completed the trial (N= 14 Bromelain; N=17 placebo). No statistically significant treatment group differences were observed (coefficient = 11.16, p=0.27, CI -8.86 to 31.18) in the primary outcome WOMAC subscales or SF-36. Both treatment groups showed clinically relevant improvement over time in the WOMAC disability subscale. Adverse events were generally mild. **Conclusion:** This study suggests that Bromelain is not efficacious as an adjunctive treatment for patients with moderate to severe OA, but its limitations support the need for a follow-up study.

PG1-09

Not on my own: Women's experience of herbal practice as participants in a randomised controlled trial

Green J[1], Hawkey S[2], Ingram J[3], Denham A[4]

[1]National Institute of Medical Herbalists, Exeter, UK; [2]School of Health and Bioscience, University of East London, London, UK; [3]Bristol Research & Development Support Unit, Bristol Royal Infirmary, Bristol, UK; [4]Department of Nursing, University of Central Lancashire, Preston, UK

Aims: To identify predominant themes in the experience of participants during the treatment process of menopausal problems by herbal practitioners. **Methods:** "Not on my own" is a nested qualitative study (Trial registration ISRCTN42406364) within "Changing with Herbs" (a pragmatic randomised controlled pilot study of the effectiveness of treatment of menopausal symptoms by herbal practitioners). Treatment consisted of a 5 month individually tailored, holistic course of treatment from 1 of 3 local members of the National Institute of Medical Herbalists, and was found to be effective. Treatment by herbal practitioners is multi-faceted and develops over time within a therapeutic relationship. To examine this complex system in greater depth, participants completed feedback questionnaires at the end of treatment. A sub-sample of 8 participants from the treatment arm was interviewed about their experiences of herbal treatment during this trial. Interviewees (mean age 57) were predominately white professionals; 3 had never previously taken herbal medicines and 5 had. Interviews were recorded, and transcripts were subject to thematic analysis by 2 researchers. This poster discusses the experience of the participants receiving a package of care from qualified herbal practitioners for menopausal symptoms. **Results:** Themes emerging of the participants' experience of treatment by herbal practitioners include: satisfaction with the treatment outcomes, holistic nature of the consultation, patient centred nature of the process, development of the therapeutic relationship, empowerment from changing behaviour such as diet, management techniques and connections with wider agencies in appropriate referral. Negative themes were few, including the taste of herbal medicine and the perceived expense were it not provided by the NHS. **Conclusion:** The treatment package from herbal practitioners for menopausal symptoms was acceptable to the participants in the study, who felt it should be a choice supported by the NHS. The whole treatment system was complex, responsive to individual need and evolved over time.

PG1-10

Effect of Revival soy on fibromyalgia symptoms: A randomized, double blind, placebo controlled trial

Wahner-Roedler D[1], Thompson J[2], Luedtke C[2], King S[2], Cha S[3], Elkin P[1], Bruce B[2], Townsend C[2], Bergeson J[2], Eickhoff A[2], Loehrer L[1], Sood A[1], Bauer B[1]

[1]Department of Internal Medicine, Mayo Clinic, Rochester, USA; [2]Department of Physical Medicine and Rehabilitation, Mayo Clinic, Rochester, USA; [3]Department of Health Sciences Research, Mayo Clinic, Rochester, USA

Aims: To evaluate whether dietary soy supplement can improve quality of life in patients with fibromyalgia as measured by the Fibromyalgia Impact Questionnaire (FIQ) and the Center for Epidemiologic Studies Depression Scale (CES-D). **Methods:** Design: Randomized, double blind, placebo controlled trial. Setting: A tertiary care center in the Midwest of the US. Population studied: 50 patients seen at a Fibromyalgia Outpatient Treatment Program and diagnosed with fibromyalgia as defined by the criteria of the American College of Rheumatology. Intervention: Randomization between daily Revival Soy shakes (20 gm of soy protein, 160 mg soy isoflavone /day) and placebo shakes (containing casein) for 6 weeks. Instruments used: FIQ, CES-D at baseline and after 6 weeks of intervention. **Results:** A total of 50 patients were recruited (49 females, median age 47.7 years); 28 patients (56%) completed the study (12 in soy group, 16 in placebo group). There was no significant difference between drop out rates in the soy and placebo groups. Reasons cited for not completing the study included GI-upset (3 patients in the soy group), bad taste (in soy and placebo group, total of 5 patients), and stress, fatigue and depression (in soy and placebo group, total of 3 patients). Patients who did not complete the study were significantly younger (median age 39.8 years) compared to those who finished the 6 week trial (median age 53.9 years) (p=0.0003). Total FIQ scores determined at study entry (SE) and at study completion (SC) decreased in the soy (SE 53.08; SC 41.93; decrease 21.2%) as well as in the placebo group (SE 60.74; SC 43.76; decrease 27.0%) (p=0.662). No significant difference in change of any item of the FIQ was noted between soy and placebo group. Total CES-D scores measured at SE and SC decreased in the soy group (SE 15.67; SC 11.67; decrease 32.9%) and placebo group (SE 20.63; SC 12.63; decrease 23.9%) (p=0.982). **Conclusion:** Revival soy and casein containing shakes combined with an educational program decrease fibromyalgia symptoms as determined by FIQ and CES-D scores. There was no statistically significant difference in the magnitude of symptom improvement between the soy and the placebo (casein) group.

PG1-11

Does St John's wort work better in German-speaking countries? Update of the Cochrane review restricted to trials in patients with major depression

Linde K[1], Schmidt K[1], Berner M[2]

[1]Centre for Complementary Medicine Research, Department of Internal Medicine Research, Technical University Munich, Germany; [2]Department of Psychiatry and Psychotherapy, University Hospital Freiburg, Germany

Aims: Whether St. John's wort extract is effective for depression is still a matter of discussion outside German-speaking countries. Several new trials have been published in the last few years. Almost all of these new trials have been restricted to major depressive disorder while older trials included patients not meeting current diagnostic criteria. For the current update we restricted our Cochrane review to trials restricted to patients with major depressive disorder. **Methods:** Double-blind randomized controlled trials comparing mono-preparations of St. John's wort (Hypericum perforatum L.) extract with placebo or standard antidepressants in patients meeting criteria for major depressive disorder were searched in PubMed, in the database of the Cochrane Collaboration Depression, Anxiety and Neuroses (CCDAN) Review Group and through contacts with experts. Selection, extraction and assessments were done by at least two independent reviewers. Pooled random effects responder ratios (RR) were calculated using RevMan 4.2.8. **Results:** 28 trials met the inclusion criteria; 17 trials included a placebo-control group, 17 compared hypericum with a standard antidepressant (6 three-armed trials). The pooled RR was 1.49 (95%CI 1.23 to 1.82) compared to placebo, and 1.00 (95%CI 0.92 to 1.09) compared to standard antidepressants. In placebo-controlled trials from German-speaking countries the RR was 1.87 (1.44 to 2.42, n=10), in those from other countries 1.07 (0.88 to 1.31, n=7). For comparisons with standard antidepressants the RRs were 1.05 (0.96 to 1.15) and 0.88 (0.75 to 1.02), respectively. **Conclusions:** Trials from German speaking countries report more favourable results on hypericum than trials from other countries. Potential explanations for these findings might be the inclusion of different patients or differences in the design and performance of trials.

PG1-12

A comparative study between Guduchi oil and Povidine-iodine as a dressing material in varicose ulcer

Dutta SC

Gomantak Ayurveda Mahavidyalaya & Research Centre, Goa, India

Background: Guduchi or Tinospora cordofolia is widely used in the diseases like erysipelas, various skin disorders, and ulcer, as mentioned in the texts of Traditional medicine of India. Povidine-iodine is widely used as an anti-septic solution for dressing in ulcer (so it has been used for dressing in control groups). **Methods:** 40 patients of varicose ulcer having no other systemic disorders eg. Diabetes Mellitus, hypertension has been taken for study. The selected patients have been divided into two equal groups. Group-1 dressed by Guduchi oil; Group-2 dressed by Povidine-iodine solution. Dressing has been done everyday for 15 days under hospitalization. The other variables in both the groups have been fixed as far as possible. Assessment based on size, growth of healthy granulation tissue formation, epithelisation, changes in smell, discharge has been done after 15 days of discharge from the hospital for both the groups in this case-control study. Results of both groups were compared by t-test. **Results:** It has been observed that Guduchi oil has better efficacy than the Povidine-iodine as a dressing material, so it has been recommended as a better alternative in dressing for varicose ulcer.

PG1-13

Prospective post-marketing surveillance study investigating an isopropanolic extract of black cohosh in tamoxifen-treated breast cancer patients with climacteric complaints

Fischer J[1], Mumm A[1], Stammwitz U[2], Bartsch HH[1], Saller R[3], Rostock M[1]

[1]Tumor Biology Center at the Albert Ludwig University Freiburg, Germany; [2]Schaper & Brümmer GmbH & Co. KG, Salzgitter, Germany; [3]Institute of Complementary Medicine, Department of Internal Medicine, University Hospital Zurich, Switzerland

Aims: The therapy of breast cancer with the anti-estrogen tamoxifen often induces or aggravates menopausal complaints. In order to provide pilot data on black cohosh in the treatment of these complaints, we conceived a post-marketing surveillance study for efficacy and tolerability of an isopropanolic extract of black cohosh (Remifemin®) in 50 breast cancer patients. **Methods:** The extract was applied 2x20mg daily for 6 months. Patients recorded their complaints before therapy and after 1, 3 and 6 months of therapy using the menopause rating scale (MRS II). **Results:** 47 breast cancer patients treated with tamoxifen, with a mean age of 56 years, could be evaluated for efficacy. 75% of the women were postmenopausal, the mean time since first tumor diagnosis was 8.6 months. At the start of therapy, in approximately two thirds of the patients, the MRS-II-total score indicated a severe symptomatology. The reduction of total MRS II score under Remifemin treatment by 4 units from 17.64 to 13.64 was statistically significant. After one month, the calculated responder rate of at least satisfactory efficacy was 68.1%, at last assessment 70.2%. Even though the therapy effect of the first 4 weeks can only be attributed to Remifemin treatment as part of intensive in-patient rehabilitation care, the persistence of this benefit over the following 5 months, without any additional therapy being applied, assures the efficacy of black cohosh extract in the treatment of the menopausal symptoms in breast-cancer patients taking tamoxifen. 90% of the women reported the tolerability of Remifemin as very good or good. 22 adverse events were reported, none of these were linked to the study medication. **Conclusions:** Within the specific collective of tamoxifen-treated breast-cancer patients with severe climacteric symptomatology, our data indicate an improvement in 2/3 of patients. Roughly 1/3 of patients did not benefit from the medication. Nevertheless, the isopropanolic black cohosh extract presents a promising therapeutic tool against the menopause-like complaints of breast cancer patients treated with tamoxifen. Randomized controlled clinical trials should further elucidate this treatment option.

PG1-14

The TU025 Keishi Bukuryo Gan clinical trial for hot flash management: Methodological barriers and lessons for traditional Asian medicine research

Radosevich DM[1], Plotnikoff GA[1,2], LaValleur J[1], Torkelson C[1], Watanabe K[2]

[1]University of Minnesota Medical School, Minneapolis, Minnesota, USA; [2]Keio University School of Medicine, Tokyo, Japan

Aims: Tests for the efficacy of TU025, a non-estrogenic Japanese Kampo herbal medicine that consists of four herbs and a mushroom, failed to substantiate successful treatment of post-menopausal hot flashes in American women. Lessons learned and recommendations for future Kampo studies are presented in light these negative findings. **Methods:** In a randomized, double-blind, placebo-controlled, phase II trial that enrolled 175 postmenopausal women, aged 45-58 years, with a flash scores greater than 28 per week, we conducted a post hoc analysis of the threats to the validity using the framework of Cook and Campbell that includes: statistical conclusion, internal, construct, and external validity. The failure to find a compelling relationship between the product and an improvement in symptoms is used to examine barriers to future Kampo studies of hot flash symptoms. **Results:** Valid inferences regarding the product's effectiveness were significantly compromised by several factors related to statistical conclusions and construct validity. First, the sample size and outcome effect was estimated based on earlier tests involving anti-depressants. This significantly overestimated the size of the therapeutic benefit of the product. Second, the primary outcome instrument, the Mayo Hot Flash Diary, proved to be unreliable. Third, the exclusion of severely symptomatic women, those under hormone replacement therapy and those on anti-depressants limited the generalisability of the findings. Fourth, the advertisement of an ancient Japanese herbal remedy and the supportive care provided during the trial may have contributed to a stronger than expected placebo response. Fifth, and most importantly, the lack of a validated instrument to determine the Kampo diagnosis of the subject's constitutional state blocked the capacity to identify and honor the traditional subgroups in which the product has historically been beneficial. **Conclusions:** Future studies of Traditional Asian Medicines must address salient issues pertaining to statistical conclusions and construct validity. Vitally needed is a validated method for determining the subject's constitutional state as well as improved measures for hot flash symptoms. In addition, given the potential referral bias for Traditional Asian Medicines, the reactivity of the experimental situation must be tightly controlled.

PG1-15

Lipolysar Long Action® is effective in reducing cardiovascular risk factors

Pisciotta L[1], Bertolini S[1], Bianchi A[2]

[1]Department of Internal Medicine, University of Genoa, Italy; [2]RENACO Srl, Crocetta del Montello, Italy

Lipolysar Long Action® is a dietary supplement based on Monascus purpureus, a fungus well known in China for its hypolipidemic activity due to its lovastatin content. When taken regularly, it can decrease the values of LDL Cholesterol by 16–25%, of triglycerides by 13–24%, and increase the levels of HDL Cholesterol by 8–14%. The dose of lovastatin taken daily with a treatment of Monascus purpureus is normally of 4.8-9.6 mg/die. It has been repeatedly noted how the action of extracts of Monascus purpureus on the haematic parameters is in fact greater than that of the corresponding dose of lovastatin, opening up the possibility that other active pharmacological substances present in Monascus act in synergy or independently of lovastatin. On the basis of this hypothesis, in the modernization process of Traditional Chinese Medicine, many companies have developed new strains of this fungus in which the action of new chemical components of the fungus has been explored. Lipolysar Long Action is one of these: with a low level of lovastatin (only 2.16 mg per daily dose) in this double-blind randomized clinical study vs. placebo, it has shown a significant effect on the group treated for TC ($p<0.002$), LDL cholesterol ($p<0.05$), triglycerides ($p<0.05$), and above all for hsCRP ($p<0.05$). The results on the hsCRP are in particular significantly higher than those obtainable with even higher doses of lovastatin, confirming the importance of new chemical components of Monascus purpureus.

PG1-16

Anti-cancer medicinal mushrooms can provide significant vitamin D2 (Ergocalciferol)

Stamets P[1], Plotnikoff GA[2]

[1]Fungi Perfecti LLP, Olympia, Washington, USA; [2]Keio University School of Medicine, Tokyo, Japan

Aims: To date, the potential pharmacologic activity of vitamin D2 (ergocalciferol) in Asian medicinal mushrooms has not been examined. This study tested the hypothesis that in mushroom species with documented anti-cancer activity, mushroom ergosterol exposure to UV-B energy from sun drying significantly increases ergocalciferol content. **Methods:** Three specific medicinal mushroom species with strain-specific documented chain of custody were grown under standard conditions indoors. Fruiting bodies were harvested and dried indoors by commercial dyers or outside under summer sun for 6–8 hours. The products were then subjected to standardized HPLC analysis in conformity with the Official Methods of Analysis of AOAC International (2000, 17th Ed). **Results:** Ganoderma lucidum (reishi), Lentinula edodes (shiitake), and Grifola frondosa (maitake) dried indoors demonstrated D2 content of 6, 134 and 460 IU per 100 grams respectively. When dried by sunlight outdoors, the D2 content increased to 2760, 21,400 and 31,900 IU per 100 grams respectively. **Conclusions:** The traditional method of sun-drying Asian medicinal mushrooms profoundly increases the availability of vitamin D2. This finding is significant because ingested ergocalciferol is transformed into cholecalciferol, a pharmacologically active seco-steroid. This binds to a specific receptor (VDR) within the superfamily of nuclear receptors that is found on nearly every tissue in the human body. VDR binding regulates gene expression for multiple physiologic functions. Cholecalciferol stabilizes chromosomal structure, prevents DNA double-strand breaks, induces cell cycle arrest, promotes differentiation, induces apoptosis, inhibits tumor invasion and inhibits tumor angiogenesis. Thus, the potential ergocalciferol content must be considered as a confounding factor in all medicinal mushroom research. This includes 1) all related beta-glucan and triterpene cancer research, 2) all contemporary clinical trials of traditional Asian mushroom-containing multi-herb formulas, and 3) all retrospective studies of diet and nutrition that use the USDA standard references (76 IU of vitamin D/100 grams of button mushrooms, 1550 IU/100 grams of shiitake mushrooms). Medicinal mushrooms have great therapeutic promise. Urgently needed is further understanding of ergocalciferol's pharmacokinetics, toxicology and metabolite biologic activity.

PG1-17

Honey as a topical treatment for wounds: Results of a systematic review

Walker N, Jull A, Rodgers A

Clinical Trials Research Unit, School of Population Health, University of Auckland, New Zealand

Aims: Popular opinion is that honey is an effective wound treatment, despite evidence from a systematic review failing to identify any beneficial effect. An updated review was undertaken to assess the effect of honey on the healing rate of acute and chronic wounds. **Methods:** Study design: Systematic review. Both randomised and pseudo-randomised trials were included. Study population: People of any age and in any care setting, who had an acute or chronic wound of any type. Primary intervention: Any honey topically applied by any means, alone or in combination with other dressing components, to an acute wound (burns, lacerations and other traumatic wounds) or chronic wound (venous, arterial, diabetic, or pressure ulcers, infected surgical wounds). Comparison interventions: Dressings or other topical agents applied to the wound. Outcomes: Time to complete healing, adverse events. Analyses: Analyses, where appropriate, were undertaken using RevMan. Where synthesis of the study results was not appropriate, a narrative overview was undertaken. **Results:** Eighteen trials including 2,015 participants were included in this review. Thirteen trials were in patients with acute wounds, one trial was in patients with burns or leg ulcers, and five trials were in patients with different types of chronic wounds. The trials were of poor methodological quality, with limited adverse event reporting. Honey dressings may be effective in treating mild to moderate partial thickness burns in comparison to conventional dressings, such as impregnated gauze, saline soaks, or polyurethane film dressings. The evidence does not support the use of honey in mixed thickness burns, minor acute wounds, or minor uncomplicated wounds left to heal by secondary intention following surgery. There is an absence of evidence to guide the treatment of chronic wounds with honey. **Conclusions:** Despite honey being used in wound management, trial evidence continues to find no clear benefit for most wound types. The poor quality of published information highlights the need for researchers in this area to publish according to the CONSORT statement. Trial registration would also help with the identification of relevant studies.

PG1-18

Recognition of Traditional Japanese Medicine, Kampo, by University hospital patients

Nishimura K, Watanabe K, Plotnikoff GA, Nobutomo I, Ito K, Sugiyama K

Department of Kampo Medicine, Keio University School of Medicine, Japan

Aims: Traditional Japanese herbal medicine, Kampo, is prescribed by physicians in both clinics and hospitals throughout Japan and is covered by Japan's national health insurance. This presentation will describe the characteristics of the patients' use of prescription Kampo medicine in one leading university hospital. **Methods:** Patients presenting June to August in 2004 to the University Medical Center Kampo Clinic responded to a self-administered questionnaire. **Results:** The survey was offered to all the outpatients and 475 responded and 435 were eligible to analysis (male; 28% and female; 72%). The primary indications for seeking care at the Kampo clinic are obstetric and gynecological problems, skin diseases and gastrointestinal diseases. The top reason why patients visit Kampo clinic is that they are not satisfied with western medicine. The main diseases of unsatisfactory treatment with western medicine are refractory skin diseases and subjective women's health concerns. Fifty-five percent of the subjects simultaneously visited a western medical clinic and took western prescription drugs (mean; 2.7 drugs). The subjects believed that it is necessary to take Kampo medicine for a long period: half of them had taken Kampo medicine for more than 1 year (average 49.3 months). Twenty-one percent of the patients had reduced the number of western medicines after Kampo medicine was initiated. **Conclusions:** In Japan, ancient, multi-herb formulas are prescribed along with modern western pharmaceuticals. Urgently needed are western-drug interaction studies, prevalence of dual herb-pharmaceutical prescribing as well as compliance studies. Such data will serve patients and physicians as well as provide preliminary data for rigorous clinical trials.

PG1-19

Systematic review on the efficacy and safety of nettle herb for osteoarthritis or rheumatoid arthritis

Chrubasik JE[1], Roufogalis B[2], Chrubasik S[1,2]

[1]Department of Forensic Medicine, University of Freiburg, Germany; [2]Herbal Medicines Research and Education Centre, University of Sydney, Australia

Aims: In Germany, preparations from Urtica dioica are in current use for the treatment of osteoarthritis or rheumatoid arthritis. The nettle herb mechanism of action is broader than that of synthetic anti-inflammatory drugs, involving inhibition of cyclooxygenase-2, lipoxygenase and cytokine release. The aim of the study was to review the efficacy and safety of treatment with nettle herb. **Methods:** Ovid (Medline), Pubmed, Cochrane Collab. Library (since 1985) and manual searching were used to identify clinical trials investigating nettle herb products in osteoarthritis or rheumatoid arthritis. The authors extracted the data on efficacy and safety independently and discussed any disagreements. **Results:** Eight clinical trials were identified; 2 were carried out with topical crude nettle leaf, one with a nettle stew 50 g/day, 5 with extracts (50% ethanol, DER 8-10:1, 1340 mg/day in n=3; 95% propanol, DER 19-33:1, 145 mg/day in n=2). Six studies were uncontrolled, one (using stew) was open controlled and one (topical leaf) had a confirmatory study design. The risk of adverse events was very low (< 1%), with rare cases of allergic skin reactions and mild gastrointestinal adverse events. **Conclusions:** It may well be that topical nettle leaf helps to alleviate rheumatic complaints. However, there is presently insufficient evidence on the efficacy of nettle extracts or nettle stew in the treatment of osteoarthritic or rheumatoid arthritic complaints. Confirmatory studies demonstrating superiority versus placebo and non-inferiority versus NSAIDs are required.

PG2-01

Prolonged cytotoxic effect of aqueous extracts from dried Viscum album on bladder cancer cells

Simões-Wüst AP[1], Hunziker-Basler N[2], Zuzak J[2], Eggenschwiler J[2], Rist L[1], Viviani A[2]

[1]Research Department, Paracelsus Hospital Richterswil, Switzerland; [2]University of Applied Sciences, Laboratory of Cell Biology, Department of Biotechnology, Wädenswil, Switzerland

Background: Bladder cancer is the sixth most common malignant disease and the ninth leading cause of cancer-related deaths. Recurrence of the superficial forms of this disease can be avoided by instillation with agents that have either a cytotoxic- or an immunomodulating-effect. Given that Viscum album (mistletoe) extracts, which are often used as an anti-cancer therapy in the complementary medicine, can lead to these two types of responses, they are likely to have potential in the therapy of bladder cancer. **Methods:** We have now focused on the cytotoxic effect of aqueous extracts of dried, entire mistletoe (Iscucin®) on bladder cancer cell lines. The effects of extracts prepared from mistletoe bushes from seven different host-trees on the in vitro growth of VM-CUB-1 bladder cancer cells was studied using colorimetric cell proliferation/viability assays. The two extracts that had the strongest cytotoxic effects corresponded to the host trees Crataegus (whitethorn) and Tilia (basswood). The lectin levels in the various mistletoe extracts were determined. While the extracts with the highest mistletoe lectin levels were relatively potent, the most effective one – Iscucin® Crataegi – had merely 61% of the maximal level detected. This suggests that other components are likely to be relevant for the observed cytotoxicity. **Results:** Further experiments included four additional bladder cancer cell lines and were performed under conditions that mimicked the instillation procedure often used in the treatment of bladder cancer. Accordingly, 2-hrs treatment with various Iscucin® extracts at different concentrations was performed. The extracts could trigger a strong cytotoxic effect, whose magnitude increased with time up to 72 hrs and persisted for at least up to 144 hrs (5 days). Again Iscucin® Crataegi turned out to be the most potent extract, followed by Iscucin® Tiliae. **Conclusions:** Our observations show that Iscucin® extracts, especially Iscucin® Crataegi, at a concentration of 8 mg/ml and more, strongly inhibit the growth of bladder cancer cells in a long-lasting way, under experimental conditions which correspond to the instillation procedure. The therapeutic potential of Iscucin® extracts in the prevention of recurrence and treatment of superficial bladder cancer will be discussed.

PG2-02

Individual patient data meta-analysis of prospective controlled cohort studies on long-term therapy of breast cancer patients with a mistletoe preparation (Iscador)

Ziegler R[1], Grossarth-Maticek R[2]

[1]Society for Cancer Research, Institute Hiscia, Arlesheim, Switzerland; [2]Institute for Preventive Medicine, European Center for Peace and Development (ECPD), Heidelberg, Germany

Aims: Mistletoe preparations such as Iscador are in common use as complementary/anthroposophic medications for many cancer indications, particularly for solid cancers. The efficacy is still controversial. **Methods:** Individual patient data meta-analysis of all published prospective matched-pair studies with breast cancer patients concerned with long-term application of a complementary/anthroposophic therapy with the mistletoe preparation Iscador. Six sets of data were available for individual patient meta-analysis of breast cancer patients, matched according to prognostic factors into pairs with and without mistletoe (Iscador) therapy. The main outcome measures were overall survival and psychosomatic self-regulation. **Results:** Overall survival was almost significant in favour of the Iscador group in the combined data set of the randomised studies: estimate of the hazard ratio with 95% confidence interval 0.59 (0.34, 1.02). Overall survival was highly significant in the combined data set of the non-randomised studies: 0.43 (0.34, 0.56). In the combined analysis of the randomised studies, improvement of psychosomatic self-regulation was also highly significant in favour of the Iscador group: estimate of the median difference and 95% confidence interval 0.45 (0.15, 0.80). **Conclusions:** The analysed studies show that therapy with Iscador might prolong overall survival and improve the well-being of breast cancer patients at all stages of the disease in a clinically relevant manner.

PG2-03

Functional competence of T lymphocytes in cancer patients treated with Viscum album extracts

Büssing A[1,4], Stumpf C[2], Tröger W[3], Schietzel M[1,2]

[1]Krebsforschung Herdecke, Department of Applied Immunology, Bochum, Germany; [2]Gemeinschaftskrankenhaus Herdecke, Tumor Outpatient Clinic, Herdecke, Germany; [3]Krebsforschung Herdecke, Department of Clinical Research, Freiburg, Germany; [4]Department of Medical Theory and Complementary Medicine, University Witten/Herdecke, Germany

Aim: Extracts from *Viscum album* (VA-E) are widely used as complementary cancer treatment. In a prospective observational study with defined inclusion and exclusion criteria we investigated the impact of 2 different dose regimes of VA-E (Iscador®) on the function of T lymphocytes from cancer patients within 6 months. **Methods:** We enrolled 71 cancer patients attending 2 different sections of a tumor outpatient clinic using different VA-E escalation schemes. Because it was not designed as a confirmatory study to prove efficacy, but as an explorative study to judge safety of dosage schemes, we had no control group. Four patients were not analyzed because they left the study within the first 3 months. We thus had 36 patients with breast cancer, 14 with prostate cancer, and 17 with colorectal tumors. 44 patients were female, 23 male. 36 patients were treated with VA-E "series packs" ("swift" escalation), 31 were intended to be treated with a "slower" escalation schema. Peripheral blood cells were taken each month within the observation period, cultured with PHA for 72 h and analyzed by flow cytometry. **Results:** Within the observation period of 6 months we observed a decline of stimulated T cell function, particularly in patients with colorectal or prostate cancer, but not in patients with breast cancer (which received lower mean concentrations per month) and not in patients with dose adaptation in response to too strong local reactions. The local reactions (as observed within the first 3 months) had no significant impact on the course of T cell function, because we observed a decline both in the group without any local reactions and within the group with strong reactions. However, the group with moderate local reactions in response to the VA-E injection had a stable course of functional T cells. **Conclusions:** An individual approach seems to be more suited, because the most stable T cell function was observed in the group with VA-E doses adaptation and in the group with moderate local reactions. With respect to the T cell function, our results indicate that in patients without local reactions, a long lasting mistletoe extract application should be paused periodically to allow T cell reactivity to recover.

PG2-04

Prescribing practices in the treatment of acute upper respiratory tract infections in complementary medicine

Jeschke E[1], Lüke C[1], Ostermann T[2], Matthes H[1]

[1]Research Institute and Community Hospital Havelhoehe, Germany; [2]Department of Medical Theory and Complementary Medicine, University of Witten/Herdecke, Germany

Aims: This study investigated the prescribing practices of medical doctors specialized in anthroposophical medicine in the treatment of acute upper respiratory tract infections (URTI) within an electronic research network. We focussed on prescribing of antibiotics, complications, recurrence rates and costs. **Material and Methods:** All prescriptions between May 2004 and May 2005 by 35 primary care practitioners in Germany were analysed. Data was extracted from practice software with special interfaces with additional linking of medications and diagnoses by practitioners. **Results:** 21,818 prescriptions for 12,081 patients (73.7% children) with 19,050 cases of acute URTI were analysed. The most common diagnosis was common cold (63.3%), followed by acute tonsillitis (12.9%). 63% were treated purely with complementary medicine. Antibiotics were given in 6.3% of cases. Predictive factors for antibiotic prescribing were the diagnoses tonsillitis (OR: 8.7) and sinusitis (OR: 2.2), concomitant disease (OR: 1.3), complications (OR: 4.3) and the specialty paediatrics. In cases that were initially treated with only complementary medicine, antibiotics were eventually prescribed in 0.7%. Overall complication rates were 0.03% and follow-up visits occurred in 6.3%. Patient had an average of 2.4 URTI/year (adults 1.7, children 2.7). Treatment costs did not differ between complementary care and antibiotics. **Conclusions:** Prescription practices in the treatment of URTI by anthroposophic practitioners were documented through the processing of routine medical data with minimal additional data. The prescription rate for antibiotics was well below the German average. Therapy conformed to guidelines and the complication rates were very low. Acknowledgements: The EvaMed project is sponsored with a grant of the SAG-Foundation and financially supported by WALA and WELEDA.

PG2-05

Long-term low concentrations of mistletoe extracts (Viscum album) Iscador® enhance the responsiveness of breast cancer cell lines

Clausing S, Eggenschwiler J, von Balthazar L, Ramos M, Viviani A

Hochschule Wädenswil, Klinische Forschung Weleda AG, Switzerland

Background: Fermented mistletoe extracts (Viscum album) Iscador® are clinically administered in increasing concentrations starting from 0.01 to 1 mg/ml within 3 weeks; then the cycle restarts at 0.01 mg/ml or the concentrations will be gradually enhanced to 10 mg/ml. **Subjects and methods:** We studied the effect of how cancer cells react when they were exposed to very low concentrations of Viscum album extracts from oak (Quercus), apple tree (Malus), white fir (Abies) or pine (Pinus) (10–5 mg/ml) for 2 and 7 weeks, and 3 months. Thereafter the IC50 of the four mistletoe preparations was determined. The experiments were performed with the three different breast cancer cell lines MCF-7, Kpl-1, and HCC-1937. **Results:** We observed a reduction of the IC50 value by a factor of 2 after pretreatment with low-dosed mistletoe extracts, mostly independent of the extract type. Except the long term cultivation with 10–5 mg/ml fermented Viscum album preparations from pine did not affect MCF-7 cells in regard of lowering the IC50. **Conclusions:** We conclude that low-level mistletoe extract concentrations are able to sensitize breast cancer cells for higher doses applied in intervals which could be more effective to overcome cancer cells.

PG2-06

The impact of the prophylactic or therapeutic application of bryophyllum on preterm delivery – a prospective study

Lapaire O, Ramos M, Zanetti-Daellenbach R, Birkenmaier A, Holzgreve W, Hösli I

Department of Obstetrics and Gynecology, University Hospital Basel, Switzerland

Aims: Preterm delivery is still the leading cause of perinatal mortality and morbidity in the western countries. Despite intensive efforts in the field of preventive care, screening and therapeutic interventions, the incidence of preterm deliveries has remained stable for over two decades. For inhibiting preterm labor, beta-mimetics have been used for over 20 years. Other medicaments with tocolytic properties include calcium antagonists, prostaglandin inhibitors and currently, antagonists of the oxytocic receptor. However, many of them show considerable side effects. Due to the stagnant long-term results of the tocolytical drugs, alternative medicaments, especially with a lower side effect profile are needed. Bryophyllum, which is produced from the leaves of Bryophyllum pinnatum, has been used since 1970 for tocolysis. However, because of its predominant use in anthroposophical clinics, trials for its evaluation have been rarely performed. Currently, in vitro studies endorsed the inhibition of myometrial contractibility. **Material and Methods:** After approval by the ethical committee of Basel and by Swissmedic, a prospective double-blind trial with orally applicated Bryophyllum versus Placebo in case of patients with preterm contractions, twin pregnancies and patients with a risk for preterm delivery, due to previous preterm contractions/preterm deliveries was started in June 2004. A total of 180 patients will be enrolled. Primary outcome consists of the extension of pregnancy. A power analysis was performed to estimate the number of included patients needed to detect a difference of one week. Secondary outcomes are rate of preterm deliveries, rate of side effects, days of hospitalization, and rate of lung maturation. At the Department of Obstetrics of the University of Basel, all multiple pregnancies will be included, as well as singleton pregnancies with preterm contractions /cervix < 25mm, or singleton pregnancies with a positive maternal anamnesis (e.g. prior preterm delivery, preterm contractions, cerclage). Foetuses with foetal malformations and intrauterine growth restriction are excluded. The trial was registered at www.clinicaltrials.gov (NCT00163579). **Conclusions:** Bryophyllum has been implemented in clinical practice not only in anthroposophical but also in tertiary obstetrical units. The current double-blind study will help to determine its effectiveness in preventing preterm deliveries in a tertiary setting.

PG2-07

Spatial and seasonal variations of viscotoxins and mistletoe lectins in mistletoe (Viscum album ssp. album) and their consideration in anthroposophical pharmacy

Urech K, Jäggy C, Schaller G

Institute Hiscia, Society for Cancer Research, Arlesheim, Switzerland

Aims: All proprietary preparations of V. album are total extracts and contain complex mixtures of mistletoe lectins (ML) and viscotoxins (VT). A crucial factor decisive for the ML and VT composition of the preparations is the seasonal and spatial origin of plant material. In the present study we measured the concentrations of ML and VT in the different organs of the mistletoe plant and followed their kinetic behaviour in the annual course of the leaves. The pharmaceutical significance of the variations is discussed. **Methods:** Representative samples of Viscum album ssp. album from Malus domestica collected twice a month have been extracted by an Ultraturrax homogenizer in 0.2 M galactose and N-acetyl-galactosamine or in 0.2 M acetic acid for the determination of ML and VT respectively. Total ML was determined by ELISA and total VT by HPLC (RP18). **Results:** In a representative 7 year old bush of Viscum album contents of ML showed a gradient from less than 1 mg/g dry weight (dw) at the periphery (leaves) up to more than 6 mg/g dw in the oldest stems. The sinker rich in lectins was devoid of VT. VT concentrations increased towards the periphery from low concentrations in the old stems up to 8 mg/g dw in the leaves. The seasonal course of total VT in the leaves showed a peak of maximal concentrations (20 mg/g dw) in June, and reached a minimum of less than 1 mg/g dw in the second year before the fall. Maximal concentrations of ML were measured in December (1.8 mg/g dw) with a subsequent constant decrease down to 0.3 mg/g dw in Mai. **Conclusions:** Dynamics of ML and VT concentrations of Viscum album in space and time suggest using defined organs of the mistletoe bush and fixed harvesting seasons to minimise variability of the plant material. June and December represent outstanding moments of ML and VT formation in the cycle of mistletoe. This points at important differences in physiological features of mistletoe in these two harvesting seasons considered in anthroposophical pharmacy of mistletoe preparations.

PG2-08

Safety and efficacy of mistletoe extract (Viscum album) Iscador® P in the treatment of equine sarcoid – a prospective, randomized, controlled, double-blind study

Klocke P, Clottu O, Spranger J, Burger D, Werner M, Ramos M, Straub R, von Tscharner C, Gerber V

Research Institute of Organic Agriculture (FiBL), Frick, Switzerland

Introduction: So far a therapy of the Equine Sarcoid (ES), a semi malignant skin tumor of equids is hardly considered as efficient. Furthermore, Sarcoids can be found as multi-focal typus or in critical localizations where success of surgical interventions is potentially very limited. Goal of this clinical trial was to evaluate in context of a prospective, randomized, controlled, double-blind study, the safety and efficacy of the Mistletoe extract (Viscum album) Iscador® P as a primary therapy of Equine Sarcoid. **Methods:** 53 horses with the histologically confirmed diagnosis ES were randomly assigned Verum (V; n=32) or Control (C; n=21). The horses received rising dosages of Iscador® P from 0.1mg to 20 mg extract/dose or physiological NaCl solution 3 times a week over 105 days s.c. The number, localization and morphology of the ES were observed and documented over 12 months. **Results:** In the Verum Group, 13 horses (41%) showed an improvement (at least 50% tumor remission). Of these cases a number of 9 horses developed a complete cure (28%). In the Control Group only 3 cases (14%; all showing complete cure) were classified as improved ($p<0.05$). While in horses with single or two ES no clear difference between Verum and Control could be found, a significantly better therapy course appeared after Verum treatment in horses with more than 2 ES: a number of 12 of 25 horses (48%) showed an improvement, 9 of these a complete remission (36%) including ES localized at the critical areas (head and around the eyes). In comparison, in the Control group only 1 of 15 cases (6%) could be classified as improved in this class. Side effects: After Iscador injections, a slight swelling could be observed in 5 of 32 cases which decreased spontaneously within few days. **Conclusions:** Iscador® P represents a safe and efficient therapy alternative in Equine Sarcoids, especially in cases with multi-focal character. In tumors grown in problematic localizations an attempt with mistletoe therapy should be conducted to avoid the risk of damage the intact surrounding tissue, particularly in the eye area.

PG2-09

Mistletoe (Viscum album) extract or vincristine? A comparative study

Kovacs E, Link S, Toffol-Schmidt U

Society of Cancer Research, Arlesheim, Switzerland

Background: Mistletoe (Viscum album) extract is used either alone or in combination with chemo/radiotherapy in the treatment of tumour patients. Vincristine is used in combination in the therapy of various tumours. IL-6 acts as a growth factor in several malignancies, including multiple myeloma. **Aims:** We investigated the effects of Viscum album Quercus (VA/Qu) extract (2000 ng lectin and 6 ug viscotoxin/ml) on six parameters in comparison with Vincristine. We used an in vitro model with five multiple myeloma (MM) cell lines (OPM-2, RPMI-8226, U-266, MOLP-8, KMS-12-BM) and one B cell lymphoma cell line (WSU-1). **Methods:** The IL-6 production was determined by ELISA, the DNA synthesis was measured by BrdU, proliferation by WST-1, the apoptosis and necrosis by Annexin-V and Propidium Iodide, the cell cycle phases using DNA reagent kit. Expression of the surface IL-6R was analysed by FACS. **Results:** None of the cell lines produced IL-6 spontaneously or after treatment with VA/Qu extract or Vincristine. VA/Qu extract inhibited the proliferation (cytostatic effect) and impaired the viability (cytocidal effect) markedly in 4/6 tumour cell lines. Vincristine had the same effect, however in all tumour cell lines. VA/Qu extract and Vincristine blocked the membrane expression of IL-6R. There was a relationship between this effect and the inhibition of proliferation. Both VA/Qu extract and Vincristine led to induction of apoptosis and necrosis. VA/Qu extract and Vincristine blocked G2/M and/or S cell cycle phases. This means, that these substances are CCS (cell cycle specific) drugs. **Conclusions:** The results present that VA/Qu extract and Vincristine act in the similar way, suggesting the use of VA/Qu extract in the therapy of multiple myeloma and some B cell lymphoma disorders.

PG2-10

Prospective randomized controlled open clinical observation over the antibiotic use reduction under the local ocular application of NaCl 0.9% plus Euphrasia eye drops versus NaCl 0.9% within 44 newborn children in the Neonatology

Stoffel L[1], Zimmermann D[2], Hunkeler R[1], Zimmermann C[1], Ramos M[3], Fathi-Torriani M[1], Nelle M[1]

[1]Universitäre Medizinische Kinderklinik, Inselspital Bern, Switzerland; [2]Universitäre Frauenklinik, Inselspital Bern, Switzerland; [3]Weleda AG Arlesheim, Switzerland

Objectives: Preterm and Term Newborn children have frequently in the first time after the birth a decreased discharge of eye secretion via tear course. Thus a secretion rope can develop, which can lead to an infection of the eyes. At the Neonatology of the Inselspital an eye infection in the Neonatal phase was treated until now with antibiotic eye drops. Due to preservative mercury it was examined in a randomized pilot project with control group the antibiotic use reduction under local ocular application of NaCl 0.9% plus Euphrasia eye drops versus NaCl 0.9%. **Patients and Methods:** The analysis took place with 44 newborn children. **Results:** Also with positive bacteriological eye results, the antibiotic use reduction with the application of NaCl 0.9% versus NaCl 0.9% plus Euphrasia with good results could be obtained. In particular, most of the cases with Staph. aureus could be treated without antibiotic therapy, since the clinical symptoms up to the arrival of the results of bacteriology had faded away clearly. A Limitation of this pilot project shows up in the diversity of the newborn children and the results of the bacteriology. In the NaCl 0.9% plus Euphrasia eye drops group the newborn children exhibited a lower birth weight, a lower Gestation age and were tendentious clinically more unstable. **Conclusion:** A therapy with an antibiotic cannot necessarily be recommended in newborn children with a positive ocular bacteriology.

PG2-11

Effective herbal tocolysis with Bryophyllum pinnatum

Rist L[1], Erni P[2], Brenneisen R[2], Ramos M[3], von Mandach U[4]

[1]Research Department, Paracelsus Hospital, Richterswil, Switzerland; [2]Lab. for Phytopharmacology, Bioanalytics & Pharmacokinetics, University of Berne, Switzerland; [3]Clinical Research Weleda AG, Arlesheim, Switzerland; [4]Dep. of Obstetrics, University Hospital Zurich, Switzerland

Background: Since the 1970s Bryophyllum pinnatum is also used as a phytotherapeutic preparation for the treatment of premature labour in the anthroposophic medicine. To characterize the effect of Bryophyllum pinnatum versus that of the conventional betamimetic drug fenoterol in human myometrium, the in vitro (ex vivo) contractility of term myometrium strips (biopsies from cesarean section, n=14) was measured. Strips were exposed to increasing concentrations of either B. pinnatum aqueous extracts or of fenoterol, each one in the absence or in the presence of oxytocin. Inhibition of spontaneous and oxytocin stimulated contractions by B. pinnatum was concentration dependent in both settings. **Methods:** To compare the tolerability and tocolytic outcome of Bryophyllum with those of beta-agonists, we conducted a retrospective clinical study. 67 pairs of pregnant women in preterm labour were treated with intravenous B. pinnatum (aqueous extract, 5%) or with beta-agonists. The pairs were closely matched for maternal age, gestational age at tocolysis, CTG recorded contractions, cervical effacement, preterm premature rupture of the membranes, and history of preterm labour. Endpoints were prolongation of pregnancy, gestational age at delivery, pre- and postpartum duration of hospitalization, maternal tolerability, neonatal outcome and morbidity. **Results:** Pregnant women treated with B. pinnatum and beta-agonists were equal in the prolongation of pregnancy (6.2 vs. 5.4 days, NS), the gestational age at delivery (38.0 vs. 37.1 weeks, NS) and the duration of antenatal and postnatal hospital stay, but had less adverse effects (34.3 vs. 55.2% with palpitation or dyspnea, $p=0.02$). The neonatal outcome and morbidity in the B. pinnatum group were equal or better (oxygen use 10.4 vs. 44.8%, $p<0.001$; respiratory distress syndrome 4.5 vs. 19.4%, $p=0.01$). **Conclusions:** Our preliminary pharmaceutical characterization of the clinically used aqueous extract of B. pinnatum revealed low amounts of the cardiac glycoside bufadienolide (ca. 66 ug/100 ml of a bufadienolide-derivative) whereas ethanolic extracts and extracts of other species contained clearly more bufadienolide-derivatives (up to 215 ug/100 ml in ethanolic extracts of B. daigremontianum). We found that B. pinnatum is save and effective in the treatment of preterm labour. A clinical study is now under way to compare B. pinnatum against actual standard tocolysis.

PG2-12

Effects of coloured light on cardiorespiratory coordination

Cysarz D, Altmaier A, Turci L, Kleinrath U, Lühr B, Edelhäuser F

Medical Theory and Complementary Medicine, University of Witten/Herdecke, Germany

Background: Bright light therapy with high intensities is known to be very effective in the treatment of seasonal affective disorders. Standardized coloured light of lower intensities showed an effect on heart rate variability (HRV). Red light led to an increase of Very Low Frequency oscillations whereas blue light led to a decrease of these oscillations. Hence, we investigated the effects of non-standardized coloured light (as used in arts therapy) on cardiorespiratory coordination. **Methods:** 17 healthy subjects (7 female, 10 male) in the age of 20-47 years (average ± standard deviation: 26.5±6.2) took part in this pilot study. They sat comfortably in armchair. (1) First they were exposed to daylight. (2) Next, they looked into a red glass which was grinded artistically on its surface. (3) Then, they were again exposed to daylight (4) followed by a second sequence of coloured light. This coloured light was blue and, again, it was grinded artistically on its surface. (5) Finally, they were once again exposed to daylight. Each sequence had duration of 10 minutes. An electrocardiogram and the airflow (thermocouple under the nose) were recorded during the whole session. 5 minutes in the middle of each sequence were analysed with respect to cardiorespiratory coordination. **Results:** Heart rate and respiratory rate did not change significantly during the whole session. The Low Frequency of HRV showed a slight increase and the High Frequency of HRV a slight decrease during the whole session. Both alterations were not associated with the exposure to coloured light. A specific effect of red light was observed in the cardiorespiratory coordination as expressed by the ratio of heart rate and respiratory rate. This ratio showed a spontaneous normalisation towards 4:1 (4 heartbeats in 1 respiratory cycle) during the exposure of red light. The blue light did not show such a normalisation. **Conclusion:** Non-standardized red and blue light showed an unspecific effect on HRV. Furthermore, cardiorespiratory coordination as expressed by the ratio of heart rate and respiratory rate spontaneously normalised during exposure to red light.

PG3-01

Effectiveness of Korean Hwang-gu acupuncture method in hypertension patients: A case report

Han C, Shin S, Choi S

Department of Medical Research, Korea Institute of Oriental Medicine, Korea

Aim: Aim of this study was to investigate the antihypertensive effect of Korean Hwang-gu Acupuncture in hypertensive patients. **Methods:** We measured the blood pressure of 22 patients who were admitted to the Brother Oriental Medical Clinic from 25th November 2005 to 27th March 2006. We included the patients only if systolic blood pressure was more than 140 mmHg or diastolic blood pressure was over 90 mmHg. The patients were treated by Korean Hwang-gu Acupuncture. To evaluate the effect of the Korean Hwang-gu Acupuncture, the blood pressure was measured before and after acupuncture treatment for a total of 4 times. Collected data were analyzed by paired t-test, repeated measure ANOVA. **Results:** After 3 weeks, there were significant decreases in systolic blood pressure ($p<0.0001$) and in diastolic blood pressure ($p<0.0019$) treated by Korean Hwang-gu Acupuncture 4 times. The effect of Korean Hwang-gu Acupuncture by measuring time on blood pressure were as follows: systolic blood pressure decreased significantly from the 1st to 4th visit but diastolic blood pressure decreased significantly after 2nd and 4th only. **Conclusion:** The results suggest that Korean Hwang-gu Acupuncture is effective in decreasing the systolic and diastolic blood pressure.

PG3-02

A study on allergic response between Bee Venom and Sweet Bee Venom pharmacopuncture

Kwon K

Department of Acup & Moxibustion, College of Korean Medicine, Sangji University, Korea

Objectives: Sweet Bee Venom (SBV) is made by removing allergen (enzyme) from the Bee Venom (BV) through gel filtration chromatography and propionic acid/urea polyacrylamide. The aim of this study was to verify allergy inhibitory action in Sweet BV in which the allergy causing enzyme is removed. **Methods:** 95 healthy adult men and women who had never received the BV therapy in the past were selected from a survey. The concentration of BV and SBV pharmacopuncture was equal at high and low dose, and the experiment was conducted under double blind conditions. **Results:** Participants of the study were 71 men and 24 women with an average age of 29.3 years. According to results of low dosage groups, SBV group showed significant reduction in pain compared to the BV group. Other allergic responses were not significant between the groups. For the high dose groups, SBV group showed significant reduction in pain, edema, itchiness and dizziness compared to the BV group. **Conclusions:** As a result of removed allergen, SBV significantly inhibits allergic responses both locally and throughout the body. This indicates wider and easier application of SBV for the symptoms applicable to the BV. Further comparative studies should be conducted to yield more objective verification.

PG3-04

Laserneedle acupuncture in dysmenorrhoea: A double blind trial

Ausfeld-Hafter B, Berger D, Kempf D

Kollegiale Instanz für Komplementärmedizin KIKOM, Universität Bern, Switzerland

Aims: The aim of this study is to investigate the effect of Laserneedle acupuncture in women with dysmenorrhoea. **Methods:** We designed a randomised double blind study with 46 female outpatients. To be included in the study the women had to be healthy, physically and mentally, without pharmacological or any kind of ongoing therapy. In addition a regular menstrual cycle with a minimum of pain intensity of 4 on the visual analogue scale (VAS) was required. Women were between the ages of 18 and 50. The computer programmed by a specialist in mathematics and statistics did randomisation automatically. The clinical part of the study took place from summer 2004 to summer 2005. The system selected 29 women for the placebo group and 17 for the verum group. Neither the test persons nor the acupuncturists, both of whom were wearing protective glasses during the therapy, knew about the group correspondence of the participants. Eight acupuncture points were selected for all participants (because eight laserneedles were available; Sanyinjiao SP6 bilateral, Taichong LV3 bilateral, Hegu LI 4 bilateral, Zhongji CV3 and Zusanli ST36 on the left side). The women were treated for 3 months, in 8 sessions of 20 minutes. They were allowed to take analgesics if the pain was very strong. The aim of the laserneedle treatment was to achieve a 50 percent relief of menstrual pain between the beginning and the end of the study comparing the range of the two highest pain levels on the VAS. For the data analysis we hired an extern institute for statistics. At the end of the study we questioned the women about changes of the menstruation cycle regarding length, bleeding characteristics, pain and related discomfort such as low back pain, constipation, and emotional disturbance for example. Information about life quality was obtained with the SF 36 questionnaire but was not analysed because subjects showed a good level from the beginning. **Results:** In this study we could not find a statistically significant difference of pain reduction between the start and the end of the study in both groups. Analysing the subjective changes of the menstruation cycle we only noticed that menstrual pain was reduced in the verum group. We also found that the use of analgesics was higher in the placebo group. Statistically these results were not significant. **Conclusions:** Acupuncture is known to reduce painful menstrual cramps. It is recognised as a therapy for dysmenorrhoea by the World Health Organisation. There is no significant pain reduction with the Laserneedle acupuncture. We think that further investigations should be done for the following reasons. There may be important limitations in our study. The degree of pain relief might be settled too high with 50 percent. A menstrual pain of 4/10 on the VAS as admission criteria might be too low. The number of women in the treatment group was not equal to the number of women in the placebo group. We did not select individual acupuncture points based on a TCM diagnosis. And last but not least many single case reports on positive effects of Laserneedle acupuncture in different diseases exist.

PG3-05

Activating effect of Siguan acupuncture treatment on inhibited-gastrointestinal motility in healthy volunteers

Oh DS[1], Jung S[1], Kim A[1], Koo CM[1], Shin SH[1], Kang BK[1], Park J[1], Ko H[1], Choi SM[1], Son CG[2]

[1]Department of Medical Research, Korean Institute of Oriental Medicine, Daejeon, Korea; [2]East-west Cancer Center, Dunsan Oriental Hospital of Daejeon University Oriental Medical College, Korea

Aims: This study was aimed to investigate the activating effect of manual acupuncture treatment at Siguan (LI4 and LR3 bilateral points) on inhibited-gastrointestinal (GI) motility through 48-hour radio-marker distribution profile in healthy volunteers. **Methods:** This study was conducted in an open, randomized, sham-acupuncture controlled, crossover study. Nineteen healthy male subjects were randomly allocated to be treated with real acupuncture at Siguan points or be treated with manual sham acupuncture as a control group. Prior to initial acupuncture treatment, GI-motility was inhibited by loperamide administrations (Arestal, Janssen), which dosing regimen was 8 mg twice a day. For radiographic GI-motility probes, subjects were administered a radio-marker capsule which comprised twenty radio-markers, and were treated with Siguan or sham acupuncture at 0 (baseline), 12, 24, and 36 hours. GI-motility was evaluated by abdominal supine radiography at 0 (baseline), 6, 12, 24, and 48 hours, as was based on the distribution of twenty radio-markers in ileum, ascending colon, transverse colon, descending colon, sigmoid/rectum, and outside the body. Defecation numbers in each subject were also monitored for 72 hours. Same procedures were performed after 2 weeks with a crossover manner. **Results:** No serious adverse event occurred in both Siguan and sham acupuncture treatment group. There were initially equivalent GI motility inhibitions between Siguan acupuncture and sham acupuncture group and similar distributive profile for 48 hours in five-above mentioned alimentary regions and outside the body. However, in Cochran-Mantel-Haenszel statistics, statistical significance was verified in 6, 12, 48 hours ($p<.0001$, $p<.0001$, $p<.05$, respectively). **Conclusions:** This study showed tolerable loperamide-induced GI inhibitory profile in healthy male volunteers, and, in non-parametric tests, Siguan acupuncture treatment ameliorated GI-motility for short-term period.

PG3-06

A new quantitative method for assessing the biological effect of minimal acupuncture using pulse information and a new type of placebo needle

Seki T[1], Sugita N[2], Yoshizawa M[3], Yambe T[4], Arai H[1], Nitta S[4]

[1]Graduate School of Medicine, Tohoku University, Japan; [2]Graduate School of Engineering, Tohoku University, Japan; [3]Information Synergy Center, Tohoku University, Japan; [4]Institute of Development, Aging and Cancer, Tohoku University, Japan

Introduction: There are few good double-blind acupuncture studies and little evidence of the effects of penetrating the skin. **Objective:** This study addressed the question of whether a new type of placebo needle and the proposed index rho_{max} will benefit the evaluation of acupuncture treatment and throw light on the characteristics of acupoints. **Methods:** Seventeen healthy subjects (10 women, 7 men; aged 31 +/- 8.2 yrs) were selected. A new type of placebo needle was used for this trial. Participants were randomly assigned into two groups. Acupuncture needles were placed on the acupoint Taichong bilaterally in supine position after a 10-minute rest with eyes open. The needles were removed after a lapse of 15 minutes and subjects had a rest for 10 minutes. More than three hours later, the subjects participated in the same trial with different type of the needle. On A group (10 patients, aged 28.9 +/- 8.3) the placebo needle was used after the real needle. On B group (7 patients, aged 33.6 +/- 8.3) the real one was used after the placebo one was used. On another day, the same trials were performed on a non-acupuncture point. The rho_{max} is the maximum cross-correlation coefficient between two signals in a Mayer wave band and is an index which shows the linear correlation of the baroreflex function. The LF/HF, the rho_{max} between heart rate and blood pressure and rho_{max} between heart rate and pulse transmission time (PTT) were calculated. **Results:** Only in Taichong the rho_{max} between heart rate and PTT declined significantly in the first half of acupuncture treatment with the real acupuncture needle. **Conclusions:** Minute needle penetration only at the acupoint changes the condition of the autonomic nervous system. The rho_{max} between heart rate and PTT has been proved to be a suitable index to evaluate the acupuncture mechanism.

PG3-07

Psychophysiological relaxation response induced by acupuncture – impact of suggestion

Bäcker M[1], Schäfer F[2], Balzer S[1], Stiegler N[1], Lüdtke R[3], Michalsen A[1], Dobos GJ[1]

[1]Chair of Complementary Medicine, University of Duisburg-Essen; Department of Internal and Integrative Medicine, Kliniken Essen-Mitte, Germany; [2]Department of Physiological Psychology, University of Wuppertal, Germany; [3]Karl and Veronica Carstens Foundation, Essen, Germany

Aims: Relaxation is believed to be a relevant therapeutic effect of acupuncture. It is widely unknown by which mechanisms this effect is mediated. In the present study we tested the impact of the needling itself, the suggestion of relaxation and the interaction of both on the psychophysiological response to acupuncture. **Methods:** 48 healthy subjects were randomised into four groups. The experiments were performed in a quiet room with subjects resting in a supine position. In group A the acupoints Ex HN 1 on the vertex were needled, group B exclusively received a verbal suggestion of relaxation, in group C acupuncture was applied in combination with suggestion and group D had to rest without receiving any intervention. Before, during and after the experiment arterial blood pressure, heart rate, electrodermal activity (EDA) and the introspective activation of the subjects (EWL self rating scale) were measured. Data were analysed by ANOVA to determine the main and interaction effects of acupuncture and suggestion on the psychophysiological parameters. **Results:** A significant decrease of psychophysiological activation at the end of the measurements compared to the baseline values was observed in all groups. Suggestion did neither have a main nor interaction effect on any psychophysiological variable. Acupuncture induced a distinct response pattern of EDA, which consisted of an initial increase during the needling and a following poststimulative decrease, which was significantly ($p<0.001$) more pronounced compared to "no acupuncture". **Conclusions:** Acupuncture appears to induce a poststimulative sympathetic withdrawal that might mediate relaxation often reported by patients directly after an acupuncture treatment. Suggestion, as applied in this trial, did not have an impact on the psychophysiological response. A relaxation response found in the "no intervention group" might reflect an unspecific effect of "simply resting" in acupuncture treatment. Further studies will be performed to investigate the response to acupuncture in patients with chronic painful conditions, who have been shown to have a reduced ability to elicit a relaxation response as compared to healthy subjects tested in the present trial.

PG3-08

A randomized controlled trial of whole-body acupuncture for tobacco withdrawal symptoms

Hyun M[1,2], Kang K[1], Koo C[1], Han S[1], Kim A[1], Jung S[1], Oh D[1], Choi S[1], Lee MS[3]

[1]Department of Medical Research, Korean Institute of Oriental Medicine, Daejeon, Korea; [2]Health Technology Planning & Evaluation Board, Korea Health Industry Development Institute, Seoul, Korea; [3]Complementary Medicine, Peninsula Medical School, Universities Exeter & Plymouth, UK

Aims: Although auricular acupuncture is commonly applied to patients who wish to quit smoking, its effect is still questionable. We investigated the effect of whole-body acupuncture and differentiation adoption to choose acupoints on the dropping of tobacco withdrawal symptoms and the cessation of smoking. Moreover, we intended to inquire the effects of differentiation-based whole-body acupuncture on withdrawal symptoms for tobacco, such as dysphoric or depressed mood, insomnia, etc. as listed in DSM-IV. **Methods:** A randomized, controlled, parallel group trial was conducted in which both patients and evaluators were unaware of the treatment. The acupoints chosen on treatment group were HT7, PC7, HT8, KI3, and KI6, and the acupoints on control group were non-acupoints, which are 1 cm-apart respectively from other acupoints, like LI12, TE11, TE12, GB32, and BL37. Six sessions of treatment were carried out over 2 weeks (3 times a week), and the participants were re-enrolled and evaluated 2 weeks after the end of 6th session. After screening 87 smokers, 80 were randomly assigned into 2 groups: 38 of treatment group and 42 of control group. 46 remained at the end of experiment. The primary outcome was Minnesota Tobacco Withdrawal Scale (MTWS), and the second ones were Beck Depression Inventory (BDI) and Beck Anxiety Inventory (BAI). **Results:** No statistically significant differences were observed in age, weight, height, BMI, their tendency of drinking alcoholic beverages, MTWS, FTND, BDI, or BAI between treatment and control group at baseline visit. Also, there were no statistically significant differences for the mean reductions of MTWS, BDI, and BAI scores from baseline visit to each visit (2, 3, 4, 5, 6, and 7 weeks) between two groups. But MTWS, BDI, and BAI showed differences within each group from baseline to each visit ($P<.05$). **Conclusions:** Since the control group that was treated with minimal non-acupoints exhibited similar consequences with the treatment group, further investigation with more thorough designs, for example, including no treatment group, is required.

PG3-09

Chemotherapy-induced peripheral neuropathy in cancer patients: Evaluation of acupuncture vs. electrotherapy vs. vitamin B – a prospective randomized placebo controlled pilot-study

Rostock M[1], Lacour M[2], Jaroslawski K[1], Guethlin C[2], Zunder T[2], Luedtke R[3], Bartsch HH[1]

[1]Tumor Biology Center at the Albert Ludwigs University Freiburg, Germany; [2]University Medical Center Freiburg, Germany; [3]Carstens Foundation Essen, Germany

Aims: Peripheral neuropathy (PNP) is an often dosage-limiting side effect of several cytostatic drugs in cancer treatment. Is a special acupuncture concept combined with electrostimulation more effective than placebo or other more usual but yet not well proved treatment options? **Methods:** Prospective randomized placebo controlled pilot-study with cancer patients suffering from PNP: electrostimulation-acupuncture vs. hydroelectric baths vs. vitamin B1/B6 capsules vs. placebo capsules. Main parameter: subjective PNP complaints (numeric rating scale = NRS) d21 - d0. Additional parameters: special PNP-score, electroneurography, common toxicity criteria (WHO), Quality of Life (EORTC QLQ-C30). Using an adaptive study-design an interim analysis (acupuncture vs. placebo) was planned after inclusion of 60 patients (one-sided t-test): A) If $p<0,0207$: acupuncture is effective, end of the study. B) If $p>0,6$: acupuncture is not effective, end of the study. C) if $0,0207 \leq p \leq 0,6$: adaptation of the needed number of patients and continuation of the study. **Results:** 60 of 199 screened patients fulfilled all inclusion criteria and were included into the study. Improvement of the subjective neuropathy complaints in the acupuncture group (NRS - mean value) was from 4,0 (+/-1,7) to 3,2 (+/-1,9) = 0,8; in the hydroelectric bath group from 5,5 (+/-2,6) to 3,8 (+/-2,9) = 1,7; in the Vitamin B1/B6 group from 4,9 (+/-1,8) to 3,3 (+/- 2,3) = 1,6; and in the placebo group from 4,9 (+/-2,1) to 3,6 (+/-1,6) = 1,3. The p-value of the difference between acupuncture and placebo group was 0,705. **Conclusions:** The proven special acupuncture concept combined with electrostimulation is not effective in treating complaints from chemotherapy-induced peripheral neuropathy in cancer patients. There was no statistical significant difference in outcome for the two other therapy groups (hydroelectric baths and Vitamin B1/B6) too, but the adaptive study design for this clinical trial was designed to answer the first question only. Further clinical research should focus on hydroelectric baths because they are used in a long tradition but are not well proved up to now.

PG3-10

A randomized, single blind clinical trial to evaluate hot flash relief efficacy and safety of Traditional Korean medical acupuncture in postmenopausal women

Kim DI[1], Roh JJ[1], Lee SD[2], Roh JW[3], Yoon SH[3], Ahn HY[4], Kim SH[5], Oh DS[6], Choi SM[6]

[1]Dept. of OB&GY, College of Traditional Korean Medicine, Dongguk Univ., South Korea; [2]Dept. of Acupuncture & Moxibustion, College of Traditional Korean Medicine, Dongguk Univ., South Korea; [3]Dept. of OB&GY, College of Medicine, Dongguk Univ., South Korea; [4]Dept of Statistics, College of Science, Dongguk Univ., South Korea; [5]Clinical Research Center, Dongguk University International Hospital, South Korea; [6]Dept. of Medical R&D, Korea Institute of Oriental Medicine, South Korea

Aims: Hot flash is a major symptom which depreciates quality of life in perimenopausal and postmenopausal women. And it has been the main goal of HRT (Hormonal Replacement therapy). As a result of the WHI study, however, benefit of HRT such as relief of hot flash was lightened by risks of that such as increase of breast cancer, endometrial cancer, coronary heart disease, cerebrovascular disease and pulmonary embolism. So many women hope to overcome their perimenopausal clinical problems with complementary medicine like acupuncture and herbal medicine. In this study we intended to confirm if proper stimulation and De qi of traditional Korean medical acupuncture could increase efficacy in hot flush relief. **Methods:** A randomized controlled, single blind study. We used two modalities of acupuncture, one with optimal stimulation and one with minimal stimulation. Same acupoints were used in both groups. 52 patients were treated twice a week for 8 weeks, and follow-up was done after 4 weeks from the last treatment. Patients checked hot flush VAS (100mm visual analog scale), frequency and duration at every visit. **Results:** Relief in hot flash with regard to VAS data was obvious in both groups. Hot flash VAS scores of study group were smaller than the scores of control group at the early stage (3rd, 4th and 8th visit), but there wasn't a remarkable difference between study and control group at the end of the trial. Besides, diminution of hot flash VAS was faster and more even in study group than control group by visualization using 'Box plot'. We compared frequency and duration of hot flash, 100mm sweating, palpitation, sleep disturbance VAS, and Kupperman Index, MENQOL, Patient's global assessment score. Both groups showed definite decrease from the baseline, but difference was not statistically significant. There wasn't any adverse event. Hot flash relief efficacy was kept in most of patients after 4 weeks' follow-up. **Conclusions:** Acupoint combination by Traditional Korean medical theory is effective in hot flashes. Superiority of optimal stimulated acupuncture therapy to minimal stimulated acupuncture therapy was not verified statistically, but hot flash relief efficacy was faster and more even in optimal stimulation than minimal stimulation.

PG3-11

Content validity of an acupuncture sensation questionnaire

Kim Y[1,2], Park J[2,3], Park HJ[1,2]

[1]Department of Meridian & Acupuncture, College of Korean Medicine, Kyung-Hee University, Seoul, Korea; [2]Acupuncture and Meridian Science Research Centre, Kyung-Hee University, Seoul, Korea; [3]Division for Research and Education in Complementary and Integrative Medical Therapies, Harvard Medical School, Osher Institute, Boston, USA

Background: Since many years subjective sensations created by acupuncture have been regarded as important components to assure that aimed intervention was properly delivered. However, a number of studies with sufficient scientific rigor on the topic is scant, albeit a few are existing. Purpose: To improve a previously tested acupuncture sensation scale, therefore to develop a better acupuncture sensation questionnaire (ASQ) by qualitative study methods in Koreans. **Methods:** We generated the items for ASQ by in-depth interviews of outpatients, constructed an ASQ through focus group discussion, and assessed content validity of the newly developed ASQ. **Results:** We interviewed 48 out-patients (age, mean (SD): 49.9 (13.4); M/F: 12/36) in Korea from August 17th to September 2nd, 2005 and from February 20th to March 3rd, 2006 The analysis of the interview transcripts provided 3 categories: the sensations during the insertion of acupuncture needle (SIA); those during the manipulation (SMA); and those while the needle is placed without any further stimulation (SM). From in-depth interviews, we initially constituted 33 items related to SIA, 59 to SMA, and 29 to SM. Following focus group discussion, in which experts constructed an ASQ comprising 60 questions (15 regarding SIA, 28 SMA, and 17 SM). From the content validity test where professional judges rated the relevance, 26 items (3 in SIA, 14 in SMA, and 9 in SM) were selected as they were rated 'relevant' in more than 70%. **Conclusions:** The newly developed ASQ, comprising 26 expressions of sensation related to acupuncture experience, is now qualified for testing construct validity and reliability.

PG3-12

Patient perspectives on acupuncture – a qualitative study

Joos S, Viveros de Moraes-Gradl O, Szecsenyi J

Department of General Practice & Health Services Research, University Hospital Heidelberg, Germany

Aims: Based on existing results of acupuncture trials it must be assumed that unspecific factors within the dynamics of the acupuncture process play an important role for treatment outcome. The aim of our study was to explore patient perspectives on acupuncture to get an idea of patient-relevant factors within the process of acupuncture treatment. **Methods:** This was a qualitative study using semi-structured interviews. We interviewed 25 patients with chronic illness who were having acupuncture treatment within the preceding 6 weeks. The interviews were recorded digitally, transcribed literally and analysed by two different researchers with ATLAS.ti software. **Results:** Key questions of the interviews comprised patients´ perceptions of the acupuncture process and of the therapeutic relationship. Furthermore, patients´ understanding of well-being, health and illness was explored. **Conclusions:** We expect that our results will help to identify patient-relevant unspecific factors within the acupuncture process and, thus, will contribute to a better understanding of acupuncture as a "complex intervention".

PG3-14

The short-term efficacy of acupuncture for chronic low back pain: Randomized sham controlled trial

Kwon YD, Lee SK, Lee JW, Jeong SK, Choi SM

Department of rehabilitation and acupuncture, Wonkwang University Hospital, Gwangju city, Korea

Aims: To determine whether manual acupuncture is effective compared with sham acupuncture for chronic low back pain (LBP). **Methods:** The inclusion criteria for subjects were LBP ≥ 3 months and age ≥ 20 years. The exclusion criteria were spinal diseases such as spinal tumor, infection and neurological deficits. The subjects were diagnosed by L-spine series and CT and randomized to two groups, manual acupuncture (MA) and minimal acupuncture (SA). MA group received manual acupuncture with De-qi used 'the method reinforcing and reducing by puncturing along and against the direction of chains respectively' on a total of 14 acupoints during 20 minutes. SA group received minimal acupuncture on a total of 14 non-acupoints during 20 minutes. Treatment was delivered three times for 4 weeks. Outcome was measured by pain intensity (VAS), Roland Disability Questionnaire (RDQ), Patient Global Assessment (PGA) at week 0, 2 and 4, and digital thermography (DT) was assessed at week 0 and 4. The primary outcome measure was change in VAS and RDQ scores between 0, 2 and 4 weeks. The data were analyzed with Repeated Measure ANOVA and ITT, and the level set for statistical significance was $p<0.05$. **Results:** 57 patients were screened and 50 patients enrolled. 25 subjects were randomized to MA group. 25 were randomized to SA group. There were three drop-outs (MA group n=1, SA group n=2). MA group had a significant decrease in VAS of 19.2±3.9 between 0, 2 and 4 weeks ($p<0.05$), and a decrease in RDQ scores of 1.2±1.0 ($p>0.05$). SA group had a significant decrease in VAS of 15.7±4.1 between 0 and 4 weeks ($p<0.05$) (not a significant decrease between 0 and 2 weeks), and a decrease in RDQ scores of 1.84±1.05 ($p>0.05$). There were no differences in VAS and RDQ scores between MA and SA groups. DT and PGA have no differences in respective groups and between two groups. Three subjects showed a side effect of fatigue (MA group n=1, SA group n=2) and there was no severe adverse event. **Conclusions:** Acupuncture is an effective and safe treatment for chronic low back pain in short-term, but acupuncture was not superior to sham acupuncture in this study. Further study including follow-up is required a rigorous research in multicenter sites. Acknowledgement: This study was supported by the Acupuncture, Moxibustion and Meridian Research Project (K06070) of Korea Institute of Oriental Medicine in 2006.

PG3-15

Effect of scalp acupuncture on language development in the rehabilitation of autistic children: An Egyptian experience

Allam H[1], Gamal El-Dine N[2], Helmy G[1]

[1]Complementary Medicine Department, National Research Centre; [2]Phoniatric Unit, ENT Department, Faculty of Medicine, Ain Shams University, Cairo, Egypt

Background: Autism is a neurodevelopmental disorder that manifests in delays of social interaction, language as used in social communication, or symbolic or imaginative play, with an onset prior to age of 3 years. Language Therapy (LT) for autistic children is the main line of rehabilitation as it stresses on its major presenting symptom; language impairment. Many autistics who acquired language (verbal) have difficulty in semantics; all of them have difficulty in pragmatics. Scalp acupuncture (scalp AP) is a modality based on the physiological function of different brain areas; where different scalp zones are stimulated with needles so as to stimulate the reflex-related nerve tissue. **Aim:** Evaluate the role of Scalp AP as complementary modality to LT in rehabilitation of autistic children. **Subjects and methods:** The study was carried out in 20 autistic children (divided into 2 equal groups A and B), diagnosed according to DSM IV classification. Age was 4-7 years (Mean 5.5 years). All were subjected to language therapy (LT) twice weekly, aiming at stimulation of cognitive and verbal abilities. Group B only was subjected to scalp AP twice weekly as a rehabilitation complementary tool (acupoints used: Du 20, 26, GV17,3 temple needles, Yamamoto YNSA:cerebrum, aphasia points: using acupuncture needles 0.3x30mm). Language test was done before and after therapy (9 months) to monitor cognition and expression (Arabic test included). **Results:** Both groups showed a significant improvement in cognitive and expressive language skills between pre and post therapy, being highly significant among group B autistics treated with Scalp Ap (attention 2.8±0.8 group A vs 3.5±0.8 group B, receptive semantics: 7±3.8 group A vs 9.4±3.1 in group B). Expressive semantics significantly improved in both groups. **Conclusion:** Scalp Ap is a successful, effective and safe complementary modality for autistic children with language disorders when combined to language therapy.

PG3-16

Physical basis of acupuncture and its neurobiological implication

Soh KS

School of Physics, Seoul National University, Korea

In the early 1960's, Bong-Han Kim proposed the existence of a new circulatory system that was the anatomical basic of acupuncture points and meridians. He claimed that the acupunctural circulation system consisted of several subsystems: the superficial systems located in the skin that corresponded to classical acupuncture system, the intravascular system existing inside the large blood and lymphatic vessels, and the organ-surface system occurring on the surface of various internal organs. These meridian-associated anatomical systems were named Bonghan ducts (BHD), and the acupoint-associated ones were referred as Bonghan corpuscles (BHC). These findings based upon the use of light microscopy and simple histological methods did not gain any further attention by the scientific community until recently. We report on the series of investigations aiming to elucidate the details of BHC and BHD anatomy and structure that has been done during recent several years. The intravascular BHDs in blood and lymphatic vessels were observed in rabbits and rats. The BHC and BHD on the inner organ surfaces were isolated and characterized by applying (1) the histological staining methods in combination with confocal laser scanning microscopy, (2) the ultrastructural analysis with scanning electron microscopy (SEM), transmission electron microscopy (TEM), cryo-SEM, SEM with a focused-ion-beam (FIB-SEM), and High voltage TEM, (3) the immunohistochemical methods to examine the cellular nature. In addition, the circulatory function was investigated by injecting nanoparticles, and Alcian blue where the measured flow speed was 0.3±0.1 mm/sec. Furthermore, the presence of chromaffine cells that produces catecholamine (adrenaline and noradrenalin) in the BHC of rabbits was confirmed by the method of biochemical (ELISA) and immunohistochemical methods. The existence of the neurotransmitter (catecholamine) at the BHC has a profound significance in connection with neurobiology of acupuncture.

PG4-01

Patient satisfaction with primary care: A comparison between conventional care and Traditional Chinese Medicine

Michlig M[1], Ausfeld-Hafter B[2], Busato A[1]

[1]Institute for Evaluative Research in Orthopaedic Surgery IEFO, University Bern, Switzerland; [2]Kollegiale Instanz für Komplementärmedizin KIKOM, Universität Bern, Switzerland

Objectives: The evaluation of patient satisfaction in Traditional Chinese Medicine (TCM) versus Conventional Medicine (COM) in Swiss primary care. **Patients and Methods:** Participants were 51 certificated TCM-Physicians, 71 COM-Physicians and 2530 adult patients. A cross-sectional observational study was performed with questionnaires aimed at fulfilment of expectations, perceived treatment effects and patient satisfaction. **Results:** Patients in Switzerland, who choose as primary care a conventional physician with additional certification in TCM have a higher chance to be completely satisfied with their treatment compared to patients who choose as primary care a physician only educated in conventional medicine. **Conclusions:** Physicians who supply TCM additionally to COM are able to satisfy the needs of their patients more completely compared to only COM practicing physicians. As explanation for that difference are to be seen the less frequent occurring side effects in TCM, a better physician-patient interaction with longer duration of consultation and different treatment expectations of patients in TCM.

PG4-02

A clinical study investigating the unjustified association of diet and acne: A rational approach from Traditional Chinese Medicine perspective

Law M[1], Chuh A[1], Lee A[1], Molinari N[2]

[1]Department of Community and Family Medicine, School of Public Health, The Chinese University of Hong Kong; [2]Department of Biostatistcs, Institut Universitaire de Recherche Clinique, Université Montpellier I, France

Aim: An association between diet and acne has long been postulated but remains unproven. Systematic review from the perspective of western medicine suggested there was not yet compelling evidence regarding the relation of diet and acne. However, the association of diet and acne is highly appreciated from Traditional Chinese Medicine (TCM) perspective. We suppose the contradiction is due to the heterogeneity in population. Susceptibility of nutritional influence might be diverse among different subsets of acne patients. In order to rationalize the paradox, the very core concept in TCM, the Yin and Yang, is introduced to differentiate the subsets. This study investigated whether certain food category associates with clinical severity of acne when we consider subjects in "Yang predominant" group and "Yin predominant" group separately. **Methods:** The completion rate of this cross-sectional study was 91.2%. 389 entrants of the Chinese University of Hong Kong, who attended their general health evaluations within a five-day duration in August 2006, were recruited randomly. Each subject's Yin and Yang score was quantified with score from –10 to +10 by four Hong Kong registered Chinese medicine practitioners, which had been shown to be a reliable method. The subject was classified as "Yang predominant" if Yin score minus Yang score was smaller than zero; as "Yang predominant" if Yin score minus Yang score was greater than zero. Diet patterns were collected by a food frequency questionnaire. Clinical severity of acne was examined by a rater who had been systematically trained and validated by a specialist dermatologist. Multivariate logistic regression was used for the statistical analysis. **Results:** After dividing the subjects into "Yang predominant" and "Yin predominant" groups, we performed the logistic regression analysis adjusting for eleven categories of food, gender, body mass index, perceived stress, sleeping hours and quality, as well as previous acne treatment. In "Yang predominant" group, fresh fruit juice (OR 1.78, 1.073 to 2.959) and dietary or soy products (OR 0.634, 0.425 to 0.947) associated with clinical severity of acne. In "Yin predominant" group, no category of food was associated with clinical severity of acne. **Conclusion:** The association of certain food categories and clinical severity of acne is justified in "Yang predominant" subjects, but not in "Yin predominant" subjects.

PG4-03

Is there a difference in the TCM-diagnosis in menopause-related symptoms between German and Chinese women? – the Shanghai-Essen-Study (SES)

Rampp T[1], Zhang L[1], Sun Z[2], Musial F[1], Dobos G[1]

[1]Chair of Complementary Medicine, University of Duisburg-Essen; Department of Internal and Integrative Medicine, Kliniken Essen-Mitte, Germany; [2]Department of Gynecology, Shuguang hospital, Shanghai University of TCM, China

Aims: Investigations comparing western and eastern populations according to menopause-related symptoms revealed a significant difference in prevalence and intensity of the symptoms, as well as in TCM diagnosis. The aim of the study presented here was to investigate possible differences between two comparable urban samples of menopausal women, one in Essen (Germany) and the other in Shanghai (China). **Methods:** Consecutive patients in the TCM-outpatient clinic of the university of Duisburg-Essen (Erich-Rothenfußer-Haus) in Germany (n=35) and in the Shuguang hospital (Shanghai university of TCM) in China (n=35), who suffered from menopause-syndrome, participated in the study. For conventional diagnostic reasons we used the Kuppermann-Index and the Menopause Rating Scale (MRS). The complete TCM-diagnosis was made by the same experienced investigator in China as well as in Germany (Z. Sun). Means were compared using Students t-test, frequency distributions were compared using Pearson chi-square. **Results:** Kidney yin deficiency was diagnosed in 17.1% of the German women in contrast to 74.3% of the Chinese women, 51.4% of the German women had kidney yang deficiency compared to 5.7% of the Chinese women. 31.4% of the German women had a combination of yin-yang deficiency compared to 20% of the Chinese women. No group differences were found for the Kupperman-Index, however, there were significant differences in specific symptoms of the Kupperman-Index questionnaire. **Conclusion:** The differences in the menopausal symptom pattern and in the most common TCM syndromes between German and Chinese women were striking. German women suffer more from kidney yang deficiency problems whereas Chinese women suffer more from kidney yin deficiency problems. Even though further research is needed, it can be speculated that different TCM-diagnosis as well as different symptom patterns in the eastern and in the western population should lead to different treatment strategies.

PG4-04

The efficacy and safety of herbal medicines for idiopathic Parkinson's disease: A systematic review

Chung V, Liu L, Bian ZX, Zhao ZZ, Fong WL, Kum WF, Gao J, Li M

School of Public Health, The Chinese University of Hong Kong

Aim: To assess the efficacy and safety of herbal medicines (HM), as a monotherapy or adjunct therapy, compared to placebo or conventional approaches in the treatment of idiopathic Parkinson's disease (PD). **Methods:** A systematic review of randomized controlled trials from both conventional and alternative medicine sources. The following databases were searched in July 05 regardless of language and publication status (1) Cochrane Central Register of Controlled Trials, (2) Medline, (3) CINAHL, (4) AMED, (5) Chinese Scientific Journal Database, (6) Traditional Chinese Medicine Database, (7) Chinese BioMedical disk (CD-ROM), (8) China Academic Journal Full Text Database, (9) China Proceedings of Conference Databases, (10) China Doctorate / Master Dissertations Full Text Databases, and (11) Database of Ongoing Trials (www.controlled-trials.com). We hand-searched a list of Chinese and English journals having the potential to include eligible papers. Outcome measures were overall improvement, quality of life, reduction of levodopa dose and adverse events. Two independent reviewers (VC and LM) assessed study eligibility and performed data extraction. Any disagreement was resolved by discussion. The final decision for inclusion and exclusion were confirmed by consultation between reviewers. **Results:** Out of 28 identified studies, nine studies were included (two written in English and seven in Chinese), each testing a different HM. Six of the trials had limited internal validity due to major flaws in design, including the lack of proper randomization; insufficient blinding; unclear inclusive criteria in terms of diagnostic criteria, baseline staging and duration of disease; lack of proper sample size calculation; and insufficient data analysis. External validity of the results was comprised due to imbalance in gender and ethnicity among the 9 included trials. No major adverse effects emerged and no specific pattern detected from the trials described such data. **Conclusions:** Besides major methodological defects, heterogeneity in 1) HM tested, 2) control treatment and 3) outcome measure hindered in-depth data analysis and synthesis. Current evidence is insufficient to evaluate the efficacy and safety of various HM. Further studies with improved trial design and reporting, with assessment on cost effectiveness, quality of life and qualitative data are warranted.

PG4-05

A feasibility study exploring the role of Chinese herbal medicine (CHM) in the treatment of endometriosis

Flower A, Lewith G, Little P

University of Southampton, UK

Aims: 1) To assess the effects of CHM in relieving endometriosis related pain and in improving quality of life over 16 weeks. 2) To help design an adequately powered, more definitive study. 3) To assess any sustained benefits in pain relief and improvements in quality of life at 24 and 52 weeks. 4) To develop appropriate research pathways and standards of good practice for future trials of CHM. **Methods:** A double blind RCT with 3 arms: an active arm (A: n=20), placebo (B: n=20) and a waiting list control (C: n=20). Comparison of Groups A and B will provide an idea of specific benefits which can be attributed to CHM, comparison of groups B andC will indicate the scale of the non-specific benefits for CHM treatment. Ethics has been obtained and recruitment is in process. Funding is available for 40 participants which, assuming a 20% drop out, requires enrolment of 48 women. Outcomes: a 10cm VAS for pain, an endometriosis specific quality of life measure (EHP 30) and MYMOP. Safety will be assessed through patient reporting and liver/renal function testing. This trial is unique in using prepared sachets of herbal decoctions which can then be matched with a placebo. This allows authentic individuated prescribing as an effective, pragmatic way of testing CHM. Statistical analysis using Analysis of Covariance will compare the placebo group with the active group when all patients have completed the blinded phase on an ITT basis. **Discussion:** The following points will be discussed: 1) The background of the trial-developing good practice guidelines for a CHM RCT using a modified Delphi technique and a narrative literature review. 2) The logistics of doing a CHM RCT within the European Community. 3) The trial methodology.

PG4-06

Quality appraisal of systematic reviews/meta-analysis on Traditional Chinese Medicine published in Chinese journals

Liu JP, Xia Y

National Research Center in Complementary and Alternative Medicine (NAFKAM), University of Tromsø, Norway

Background: Systematic review is considered as high level of evidence for evaluating health care interventions. In order to understand the available research evidence on traditional Chinese medicine (TCM), we critically appraised the quality of reports of systematic review/ meta-analysis on TCM published in Chinese journals. **Methods:** We searched Chinese electronic full-text databases including CNKI, VIP and Wanfang to identify the reports of systematic reviews or meta-analyses on TCM including herbal medicine, acupuncture and moxibustion, as well as integrated traditional and western medicine. We used a self-developed data extraction form based on 18 items from QUOROM (quality of reporting of meta-analyses) Statement plus information on diseases reviewed, databases searched, the journals that published the reviews. The main components extracted were title/abstract, objectives, source of data, quality assessment of the included studies, methods of data extraction and data synthesis. **Results:** 82 systematic reviews on TCM were published in Chinese journals between 1998 and May 2006, three reviews were published twice, and 79 reviews were included for appraisal. 51 different diseases were reviewed, mainly focusing on cardio-vascular diseases, metabolic and endocrine diseases, GI diseases, etc. The 82 reviews were published in 45 Chinese journals. Almost all reviews included randomised clinical trials mainly targeting on Chinese herbal medicine (50 reviews), acupuncture (9 reviews), and integrative medicine (4 reviews). Among them, 10 reviews were registered as Cochrane reviews (The Cochrane Library, Issue 2, 2006). 27 reviews (34%) searched exclusively Chinese databases and 37 reviews (47%) had additional manual searches for the included studies. 53 reviews (67%) assessed methodological quality of the included studies. There was insufficient description of the study selection, data abstraction and analyses. None of the reviews used flow chart to describe the process of selection, inclusion and exclusion of studies. **Conclusions:** Few reviews reached international standard of reporting of meta-analyses and the insufficient description of methodology for conducting systematic reviews may bring about biases. Advance training for the reviewers is warranted.

PG4-07

Antioxidant activity of extracts from six Chinese herbal medicines

Lu Y[1,2], Merzig MF[2], Jenett-Siems K[2], Qingguo W[1]

[1]Beijing University of Chinese Medicine, Beijing, China;
[2]Institut für Pharmazie, Freie Universität Berlin, Germany

Aim: Oxygen radicals play well-established roles in many diseases such as cancer, atherosclerosis and dementia. They can cause DNA damage, oxidation of proteins and lead to the cell death. In our study, 6 herbal remedies which are used in traditional Chinese medicine for treating dementia were studied to investigate their superoxide scavenging activity and the inhibition of xanthine oxidase activity. **Methods:** These 6 herbs were extracted with methanol and then partitioned between dichloromethane, ethyl acetate and water respectively. **Results:** The results showed that 3 herbs, Cynomorium songaricum Rupr. Coptis chinensis Franch. and Scutellaria baicalensis Georgi had an antioxidative effect. The methanol extracts of Cynomorium songaricum and Coptis chinensis were effective in scavenging superoxide anions generated by the xanthine-xanthine oxidase system (OX/XTT) (IC_{50}=21.2 μg/ml and 22.54 μg/ml respectively) without inhibiting the formation of uric acid. The dichloromethane extract of Scutellaria baicalensis inhibited uric acid formation by xanthine oxidase as well as formation of superoxide anions in the OX/XTT system (IC_{50}=3.04 μg/ml and 13.76 μg/ml respectively). **Conclusion:** The results demonstrated that the different extracts were able to interfere through different ways with the superoxide anion generation. Thus, it can be assumed that the 3 Chinese herbs may contribute to reduce the risk of diseases induced by superoxide through their antioxidant activity.

PG4-08

Chinese herbal medicine for diabetic foot ulcers: A systematic review on randomized controlled trials

Liu JP, Zhang J

National Research Center in Complementary and Alternative Medicine (NAFKAM), University of Tromsø, Norway

Background: Diabetic foot ulceration is one of the common complications of diabetic patients. Chinese herbs have been used for treating diabetic foot and clinical trials have been published. **Objective:** To assess the efficacy and safety of Chinese herbs in patients with diabetic foot. **Methods:** Protocol of the systematic review was published in the Cochrane Library in 2006. We searched the Cochrane Wounds Group Specialized Register, Medline (1966 to 04/2006), Embase (1974 to 4/2006), Chinese Biomedical Database (1979 to 4/2006), CNKI (1994 to 5/2006), and VIP (1989 to 5/2006) to identify randomized clinical trials

(RCTs) regardless of language and publication status. We also hand searched 10 Chinese journals. The inclusion criteria were RCTs or quasi-RCTs testing Chinese herbal medicine in patients with diabetic foot ulcer. Primary outcome included clinical symptoms (heal of ulcers, numbness and pain). Two authors extracted data independently, and assessed the quality using Jadad scale plus allocation concealment. **Results:** 30 RCTs and 1 quasi-RCT were included involving 2061 patients in total. They were all published in Chinese and the quality of the trials is low (Jadad Scale 1 score). No trial used blinding or placebo. Meta-analyses showed that supplementing qi and nourishing yin (SQNY) herbs and heat-clearing and detoxifying (HCD) herbs improved ulcer healing over 80% and disappearance of numbness and pain compared with conventional therapy (RR of SQNY 0.62 [95%CI 0.47–0.81] from 3 trials, and RR of HCD 0.57 [0.37–0.88] from 3 trials). For outcome of reducing amputation rate, herbs of SQNY, HCD, and promoting tissue regeneration were better than conventional therapy, and the RR was 0.27 [0.16–0.46], 0.33 [0.18–0.62], and 0.27 [0.19–0.40], respectively. The reported adverse effects were skin itching, blood stasis in skin, vomiting and dry mouth. **Conclusions:** The evidence from small and low quality trials is not sufficient to recommend Chinese herbal therapy for diabetic foot ulcer. Large, rigorously designed trials are warranted.

PG4-09

Effectiveness of Traditional Chinese Medicine in primary care

Wong W, Lam Lo Kuen C, Fong LK, Li Z, Fai LK

Family Medicine Unit, The University of Hong Kong, China

Background: Traditional Chinese medicine (TCM) is commonly used in primary care in Hong Kong, but research evidence on the effectiveness of TCM in primary care is lacking. The aim of the present study is to determine the effectiveness of TCM in primary care. **Objectives:** To evaluate whether TCM consultation can significantly improve the quality of life of patients in primary care; to find out whether there was any difference between the different TCM disciplines; and to explore any correlation between patient's subjective assessment and TCM practitioner's objective evaluation. **Methods:** A prospective, longitudinal study on 387 consecutive new patients who consulted the internal medicine, bone-setting and acupuncture TCM primary care outpatient clinics in Tung Wah Hospital in Hong Kong. All new patients attending the study outpatient clinics were recruited. Each subject was asked to complete a structured questionnaire on socio-demography, morbidity and service utilization, the Chinese Quality of Life instrument -HK version (ChQoL-HK) and the Chinese (Hong Kong) SF-36 (SF36-HK) before the consultation with the TCM practitioner. Each subject was followed up two weeks later at the clinic when he/she was re-assessed by the TCM practitioner and was asked to complete the ChQoL-HK and SF36-HK again, and a global rating on change of the condition. Those who could not return to the clinic were followed up by telephone. Outcome Measures: The primary outcome measure was the change in scores in HRQoL measured by the ChQoL-HK and SF36-HK after the TCM consultation. The secondary outcome measures were the subjects' global rating and the TCM practitioner's objective evaluation on improvements. The outcomes of patients attending the three TCM clinics were compared. The ChQoL and SF36 scores were correlated with the TCM practitioner evaluation and the patients' global rating of change. **Results:** The majority (69%) of subjects consulting the primary care TCM clinics had musculo-skeletal symptoms/ complaints (TCM diagnosis of Meridian and limb syndrome) while 12% had upper respiratory tract infections (TCM diagnosis of external syndrome). One third of the subjects had not used other health services before consulting the TCM clinics. All domain mean scores of ChQoL-HK and SF36-HK of subjects of all three (internal medicine, bone-setting and acupuncture) primary care TCM clinics improved significantly two weeks after the consultations. The greatest improvement was found in the physical-health related domains. The improvement was significantly greater among subjects consulting the bone-setting and internal medicine clinic than acupuncture clinics. 74% of subjects reported an improvement in their global rating of change in their condition, and 54% of the subjects were rated by the TCM practitioners to have improved. There were significant correlations between changes in HRQoL scores with patient's global rating but not with TCM practitioner's assessment. **Conclusions:** Many subjects consulting TCM as the sole and first primary care service. Musulo-skeletal symptoms/complaints were the most common reason for consultation, which are different from the morbidity patterns presenting to TCM specialist clinics and Western medicine primary care services, suggesting that they serve different patient needs. TCM consultations were associated with significant improvement in Quality of Life of patients. HRQoL as a subjective outcome measure complements the objective assessment of TCM practitioners on the effectiveness of treatment. Further research with longer follow-up period is needed to examine the long-term HRQoL outcome of TCM treatments, and comparative studies between the effectiveness of TCM and Western Medicine primary care services will be useful for informing the public on their relative roles in our health care system.

PG4-10

Effect of YunZhi and Danshen in post-treatment breast cancer patients

Wong ELY, Wong CK, Lam CK, Fong C, Leung PC

The Nethersole School of Nursing & School of Public Health, The Chinese University of Hong Kong

Aims: Breast cancer is the most common cancer in women worldwide. Discomfort, fatigue and poor quality of life are usually arisen from the anticancer treatments including surgery, chemotherapy, radiotherapy, hormonal therapy, or combination therapy, because of the suppressed immunological function. YunZhi (Coriolus versicolor) and Danshen (Salvia miltiorrhiza) has been shown to benefit the immunology. To promote the immune system and hence to enhance the quality of life in the breast cancer patient; therefore, immunomodulatory activities of YunZhi may have potential benefits on quality of life, and is compatible with chemotherapy and radiation therapy of cancer. This study aimed to evaluate the oral consumption of the combination formula of YunZhi and Danshen on the quality of life in post-treatment breast cancer patients. **Methods:** A Longitudinal study design in breast cancer patients was used in the study. Breast cancer patients who were female; age 30-65; stage I to III breast cancer based on TNM Classification and the American Joint committee on Cancer (AJCC) stage groupings; completion of anticancer treatment within the last 3 years; normal liver and renal function would receive 6-month YunZhi and Danshen combination capsule on daily basis. Participants would be assessed at baseline, month 2, month 4 and month 6 using SF-36 quality of life questionnaire and vitality questionnaire. Adverse events were also monitored. The breast cancer subjects were recruited from two local hospitals. Univariate analysis for repeated measurements was used for the evaluation of changes in the quality of life and vitality. **Results:** Eighty-two breast cancer patients were recruited and three withdrew from the study due to the complaint of frequent follow-up. No serious adverse effect was reported in the whole study period of all participants. The results of the parameters for SF-36 quality of life indicated that physical function, role-physical, role-emotion, and health transition were significantly increased ($p<0.05$) upon the 6-month YunZhi-Danshen regimen. Moreover, the parameters of vitality including fatigue level, sleeping pattern, appetite, bowel movement, and emotional status were significantly improved ($p<0.001$) in breast cancer patients after taking YunZhi-Danshen capsules. **Conclusion:** The regular oral consumption of YunZhi-danshen capsules could be beneficial for promoting the quality of life in post-treatment breast cancer patients.

PG4-11

Supplementary treatment with herbal medicine on SARS or SARS-like infectious diseases: A randomized, double-blind and controlled preliminary trial

Hsu CH[1,6], Hwang KC[2], Chao CL[3], Chang SGN[4], Ho MS[5], Chou P[6]

[1]Department of Chinese Medicine, Taipei Hospital, Taiwan; [2]Department of Pediatrics, Taipei Hospital, Taiwan; [3]Department of Chest Medicine, Taipei Hospital, Taiwan; [4]Department of Radiology, Taipei Hospital, Taiwan; [5]Institute of Biomedical Sciences, Academia Sinica, Taipei, Taiwan; [6]The Community Medicine Research Center and Institute of Public Health, National Yang-Ming University, Taipei, Taiwan

Background/Aims: In view of the possible beneficial effect of natural herbal medicine (NHM) on SARS, we conducted this study to examine whether NHM is of any benefit as a supplementary treatment of SARS or SARS-like infectious disease. **Methods:** This was a randomized, double-blind, placebo-controlled trial conducted in Taipei Hospital, Taiwan 2003. A total of 28 patients fulfilled the WHO inclusion criteria and our exclusion criteria. All enrolled patients received routine western-medicine treatment. Patients were randomly assigned to one of the three supplementary treatment groups: NHM A (n=9), NHM B (n=9), or placebo (n=10). Every patient took chest X-ray every one or two days. Reading radiologists set up a standard 0 to 3 scoring system according to the severity of infiltration in each lung field (three lung fields in both right and left lungs). The main outcome measurements were the improving chest radiographic scores and the duration (days) till improvement (DI). The prognosis was also evaluated. **Results:** One patient from the placebo group passed away. NHM A took less days before showing improvement (6.7±1.8 days) compared with placebo group (11.2±4.9 days), which showed statistical significance ($p<0.05$). **Conclusions:** The initial results showed that supplementary treatment with NHM A shortened DI compared with the control group, which might be the possible favourable benefits. The findings need to be verified with a larger sample.

PG4-12

Tai Chi for cardiovascular disease and its risk factors: A systematic review of randomized clinical trials

Lee MS[1], Pittler MH[1], Taylor-Piliae R[2], Shin BC[3], Kong JC[3], Ernst E[1]

[1]Complementary Medicine, Peninsula Medical School, Universities of Exeter & Plymouth, Exeter, UK; [2]Stanford Prevention Research Center, Stanford University School of Medicine, CA, USA; [3]Department of Oriental Rehabilitation Medicine, Wonkwnag Univerity, Iksan, South Korea

Aims: The aim of this systematic review is to assess the clinical evidence of tai chi for cardiovascular diseases and its risk factors. **Methods:** Eighteen electronic databases were searched up to August 2006 without language restriction. Randomised clinical trials (RCTs) testing tai chi and assessing clinically relevant outcomes in human patients with cardiovascular disease and its risk factors regardless of control interventions were considered. The selection of studies, data extraction and validation were performed independently by two reviewers. Methodological quality was evaluated using the Jadad score. **Results:** One hundred and seventy five potentially relevant studies were identified and 7 RCTs could be included. Four RCTs were identified for hypertension and one RCT for each of acute myocardial infarction, stroke and chronic heart failure. Trials assessing hypertension demonstrated greater blood pressure reduction in the tai chi groups compared with controls. The meta-analysis showed a significant effect of tai chi compared with no treatment in patients with hypertension [weighted mean difference (mmHg), systolic blood pressure -21.5, 95% confidence interval -25.8 to -17.1, $p<0.001$; diastolic blood pressure -12.1, 95% confidence interval -15.4 to -8.8, $p<0.001$]. Compared to aerobic exercise there were no significant differences for systolic and diastolic blood pressure. **Conclusion:** The evidence of tai chi for treating cardiovascular diseases and its risk factors is scarce. For hypertension the evidence is encouraging suggesting potential effectiveness.

Acknowledgment: MS Lee was supported by the Korean Research Foundation Grant (M01-2005-214-10334-0).

PG4-13

Assessing morphological characteristics within traditional Chinese tongue diagnosis – a reliability study

Li Y, Linde K, Dai J, Zhang J, Hager S, Melchart D

Centre for Complementary Medicine Research, Technical University Munich, Germany

Background: The assessment of the patient's tongue is a crucial diagnostic tool in traditional Chinese medicine. However, the reliability and validity of tongue diagnosis has rarely been investigated. As a first step in what we hope will develop to a series of studies on tongue diagnosis we investigated the reliability of the assessment of morphological characteristics. **Methods:** A random sample of digital tongue photographs from 101 patients was taken from a larger database in a hospital for traditional Chinese medicine in Kötzting, Germany. Three (two Chinese, one German) physicians with extensive experience in tongue diagnosis independently assessed 14 morphological items selected after two small pilot series. Inter-rater reliability was assessed with Cohen's kappa (classification of agreement: <0.40 poor, 0.40 to 0.59 moderate, 0.60 to 0.74 good, >0.74 excellent). **Results:** Kappa-values for the 14 items (× three pairs of raters = 42 kappa values) covered a broad range from 0.17 to 0.89. Agreement was classified as poor in 12 comparisons, as moderate in 20, as good in 4 and as excellent in 6 comparisons. Items with good or excellent agreement for all three pairs of raters were teeth prints and colour of tongue coating. Raters often disagreed whether spots were present (kappa < 0.40). Assessments of colour showed low to moderate agreement, assessments of the type of tongue coating were highly variable. **Conclusions:** In this study agreement in the assessment of morphological characteristics of the tongue between three experienced raters was highly variable. Assessments were performed under "clinical conditions" with limited standardized instructions for decisions. Agreement could probably be increased considerably with intense standardization; however, this does not seem to reflect normal clinical conditions.

PG4-14

A systematic review on use of Chinese herbal medicine for primary dysmenorrhoea

Zhu X[1], Proctor ML[2], Bensoussan A[3], Wu E[4]

[1]University of Western Sydney, Australia; [2]Cochrane Menstrual Disorders and Subfertility Group, Department of Obstetrics & Gynaecology, Auckland University, New Zealand; [3]University of Western Sydney, Australia; [4]Private Chinese medicine practitioner in Sydney, Australia

Aim: This review aims to compare randomised controlled trials of Chinese herbal medicine as treatment for women with primary dysmenorrhoea to establish the efficacy and safety of Chinese herbal medicines. **Methods:** The databases both in English language were searched. The attempt of searches was to identify 58 relevant randomised controlled trials (RCTs). All trials were assessed for methodological quality using the Jadad Scale. Statistical analysis was performed using the Review Manager software. **Results:** The main results were: 1) Chinese herbal medicine might have significant therapeutic effect, 2) Compare to NSAIDs, Chinese herbal medicine had long term effect, and 3) Chinese herbal medicine had a lower level of adverse effect to conventional treatment. Nevertheless, there are concerns about the quality of the trials. The majority of trials demonstrated the effectiveness of Chinese herbal medicine in comparison with western drug or placebo. Publication bias might be an explanation. The method of randomization was inadequately described. Placebo was seldom used. The outcomes measures were inadequately defined. Statistic analysis was weak. **Conclusion:** The available information on use of Chinese herbal medicine suggests it is effective for primary dysmenorrhea as anecdotal experience indicated. There is insufficient evidence to determine the effectiveness of Chinese herbal medicine in reducing dysmenorrhea in comparison with NSAIDs, but the favourable result is the long-term effect from Chinese herbal medicine. Overall, careful design and conduct of the trial such as a randomized controlled trial of Chinese herbal medicine with a larger number of participants will provide better evidence of the value of Chinese herbal medicine.

PG5-01

Growth stimulation of dwarf peas (Pisum sativum l.) through homeopathic potencies of gibberellic acid

Majewsky V[1], Heuwieser W[2], Klocke P[1], Baumgartner S[3,4]

[1]Research Institute of Organic Agriculture FiBL, Frick, Switzerland; [2]Clinic for Reproduction, Faculty of Veterinary Medicine, Berlin, Germany; [3] Institute for Complementary Medicine KIKOM, University of Bern, Insel-Spital, Bern, Switzerland; [4]Society for Cancer Research, Institute Hiscia, Arlesheim, Switzerland

Aims: In earlier investigations with dwarf peas (Pisum sativum L.) specific effects of homeopathic potencies of plant growth substances on pea shoot growth were observed. The effect size of the homeopathic potencies seemed to weaken during the course of the experiments. This study aimed at analysing critical factors modulating the response of the pea system, such as seed quality, conducting person, and date of the experiments. **Methods:** 17 batches of dwarf pea seed of different seed quality were tested. Special attention was paid to the stage of maturation at time of harvest. The potencies gibberellic acid 17x and 23x and a series of potency levels (17x–24x) were tested against two controls, distilled water and succussed distilled water. Pea seeds were immersed in potencies of gibberellic acid or water controls for soaking for 24 hours. Peas were planted in a standard cultivation substrate and grown for 14 days under controlled laboratory conditions. Shoot length was measured after harvesting, data were analysed with analysis of variance (ANOVA). All experiments were randomised and blinded. **Results:** In 3 out of 17 seed batches, effects on pea shoot growth could be observed for certain potency levels of gibberellic acid. 17x and 23x - Batch 8: 17x tended to decrease growth (Fisher LSD-Test: $p<0.004$; F-Test: $p<0.1$); Batch 9: interaction between potency treatment and date of experiment (F-Test: $p<0.003$). 17x - 24x - Batch 5: growth stimulation through 17x and 18x (F-Test: $p<0.04$); Batch 9: interaction between potency treatment and date of experiment (F-Test: $p<0.0002$). **Conclusions:** Homeopathic potencies of gibberellic acid influenced growth of dwarf peas. The response of the system depended on factors of seed quality and other still unknown conditions. Immaturity of seed seemed not to be the only decisive factor rendering the seed sensitive to potencies of gibberellic acid. Because of the varying response of the test system, this plant model is not yet appropriate to study questions of homeopathic pharmaceutics in detail.

PG5-2

Duckweed (Lemna gibba L.) as test organism to investigate effects of potentised substances

Scherr C[1], Simon M[2], Spranger J[1], Baumgartner S[3,4]

[1]Research Institute of Organic Agriculture, Frick, Switzerland; [2]Institute for Chemistry and Biology of the Marine Environment ICBM, University of Oldenburg, Germany; [3]Institute of Complementary Medicine KIKOM, University of Bern, Switzerland; [4]Society for Cancer Research, Institute Hiscia, Arlesheim, Switzerland

Aims: Homeopathic remedies have been used for more than 200 years. Specific effects of these pharmaceuticals are often questioned, however, since their mode of action is still unknown. The aim of this study was to develop a stable and reliable test system to investigate effects of potentised substances on the growth rate of a small, fast growing water plant, using duckweed (Lemna gibba L.), as test organism. **Methods:** In a screening twelve substances, including unspecific and specific toxins, nutrients, plant hormones and homeopathic remedies, were tested in a potency range of 14x to 30x. In the main experiments 5–6 independent replications of potency series of several substances were performed. Duckweeds were grown in beakers (n=100) under controlled light and temperature conditions in a plant growth chamber. Five replicates (beakers) of controls and potencies, respectively, were included in each experiment. During seven days leaf area and leaf number were measured five times using a non-destructive image analysis method. The growth rate was calculated for different time courses. Statistical analysis was based on analysis of variance (ANOVA) F tests. All experiments were randomised and blinded. **Results:** Variability of the test system was assessed in water-control-runs (systematic negative controls) with water as the only test substance. The test system was stable and accurate with coefficient of variance of 3–4%. False positive results could be excluded. Out of four test substances selected from the screening gibberellic acid had the most pronounced effect in the replication experiments; potency levels 15x, 17x and 23x significantly and reproducibly reduced the growth rate of Lemna gibba ($p<0.03$). For potentised kinetin and argentum nitricum we observed significant interactions ($p<0.05$ and $p<0.01$, respectively) between treatment and experiment number, indicating specific potency effects modulated by still unknown factors. **Conclusions:** We observed specific effects of potentised substances on the growth rate of Lemna gibba. This observation supports the use of homeopathic potentisation to produce specific remedies.

PG5-04

Observational prospective study of homeopathic treatment in patients with migraine, attending the headache clinic of "G. Gennimatas" Athens General Hospital

Kivellos S, Papatriantafyllou J, Papilas K, Vithoulkas G, Karagerorgiou K

International Academy of Classical Homeoapthy, Alonissos, Greece, and Headache Clinic & Neurology Department, Athens General Hospital "G.Gennimatas", Athens, Greece

Background and aims: Homeopathy trials of migraine prevention have yielded inconclusive results, partly due to different practice among various schools. We performed an observational prospective study of classical homeopathy in patients attending the Cephalalgia Clinic. **Methods:** Forty-two consecutive patients who attended the clinic while one of the authors was available were assigned to receive homeopathic treatment, according to the principles recommended by the I.A.C.H. and G.Vithoulkas. Additional evaluation by a neurologist was performed at baseline, 6 and 12 months. Primary and secondary measures of migraine severity and impact on quality of life were recorded and analyzed. **Results:** Thirty-six patients opted only for homeopathic treatment until the completion of the study, aged (mean±SD) 34±12 years, with a baseline HIT-6 score of 65±4. Significant improvement was recorded at 6 months (HIT-6 48±8, $p<0.0009$ vs baseline, Wilcoxon signed ranks test), which was further established at 12 months (HIT-6 41.2±7, $p<0.0009$ vs 6-months). Eighteen patients had been previously administered TCAs or antiepileptics for sufficient time without remarkable improvement. A difference in HIT-6 score between those 'resistant' to previous therapy and 'new' patients was found at six months (51.5±7 vs 44.5±7, respectively, $p<0.01$, Mann-Whitney test), but not at baseline (66±3.8 vs 64±4, respectively) or after 12 months (41.6±8 vs 40.6±5.3, respectively). Migraine severity (VAS) decreaed by 72% and frequency by 81% at 12 months ($p<0.0001$ for both comparisons vs baseline). Mood was consistently higher at 12 months (Verbal Analogue Scale, $p<0.001$). Observed potential adverse effects on all 42 patients were an initial 'aggravation' of migraine symptoms in 69%, recurrence of past medical diseases (e.g. infections, eczema) in 33%, temporary emotional instability in 59% of the patients. **Conclusion:** These results compare favorably with other modalities of migraine treatment. Therefore, homeopathy, as applied in this context, warrants further research with appropriately designed RCTs.

PG5-05

Long-term outcome in a prospective observational study in patients treated with classical homeopathy

Witt CM[1], Mengler N[1], Lüdtke R[2], Willich SN[1]

[1]Institute for Social Medicine, Epidemiology and Health Economics Charité University Medical Center, [2]Karl and Veronica Carstens Foundation, Germany

Aims: Very little is known on the long-term outcome in patients who chose to receive homeopathic medical treatment. We investigated homeopathic practice in an industrialized country under everyday conditions. **Methods:** In a prospective, multicentre cohort study with 103 primary care practices with additional specialization in homeopathy in Germany and Switzerland, data from consecutive consulting the physician for the first time were observed. The main outcome measures were: Patient assessments (numeric rating scales from 0 to 10 for disease severity and SF 36 for quality of life) at baseline, and after 3 months, 1, 2 and 7 years. This analysis focuses on the 7 years follow-up. **Results:** From a total of 3677 patients 2690 (1871 adults (27% men, mean age 50.5 ± 12.3 years; 73% women, 47.7 ± 11.9 years) and 819 children (52% boys, 13.8 ± 4.0 years; 48% girls, 14.4 ± 4.3 years) completed a standardized questionnaire. Ninety-seven percent of all baseline diagnoses were chronic with an average duration of 8.8 ± 8.0 years. Disease severity decreased significantly ($p<0.001$) between baseline and 7 years (adults from 6.1 ± 1.7 to 2.7 ± 2.6; children from 6.1 ± 1.8 to 1.7 ± 1.9). For adults improvements were observed for quality of life (Physical Component Score from 46.9 ± 9.8 to 51.0 ± 9.1 and Mental Component Score from 39.5 ± 11.7 to 47.2 ± 10.3, $p<0.001$ for both respectively). **Conclusions:** After 7 years disease severity and quality of life demonstrated marked and sustained improvements following homeopathic treatment period. Our findings indicate that homeopathic medical therapy may play a beneficial role in the long-term care of patients with chronic diseases.

PG5-06

Lindan-suppressed wound healing re-established by Traumeel S – studies with hepatocytes, granulocytes and hepatic stellate cells in a newly developed in vitro model

Gebhardt R, Köhnke D

Department of Biochemistry, University of Leipzig, Leipzig, Germany, Biologische Heilmittel Heel GmbH

Introduction: Traumeel S is a modern homeopathic combination preparation commonly used in the treatment of trauma, inflammation and degenerative processes (i.e. tendon injuries, sprains, contusions, effusions). Several clinical trials and biochemical evaluations confirm the efficacy or rather give an idea for the mode of action of the preparation. In order to examine matrix stabilizing and toxin neutralizing properties of the remedy, its effect on Lindan-suppressed wound healing was analysed by means of a newly developed in vitro model. **Methods:** Using transfilter wells with hepatocytes cultured on a specialized extrazellular matrix (ECM) a sophisticated in vitro model was developed allowing evaluation of the influence of Traumeel S on complex effects of environmental chemicals such as Lindan. These included granulocyte induced degradation of the ECM, the liberation of Lindan and its harmful influence on hepatic stellate cells (HSC) determined by a wound-healing assay. **Results:** I. The developed in vitro model proved suitable to analyse protective properties of Traumeel S. II. Traumeel S was found to re-establish wound healing suppressed by Lindan, when it was present after addition of granulocytes, i.e. during liberation of Lindan and during the wound-healing assay. **Conclusion:** The results show that Traumeel S is capable to affect complex physiological processes which are involved in toxin neutralisation and wound healing. The protective effect of Traumeel S against Lindan is in line with basic concepts of homotoxicology and may be due to several reasons: (a) reduced degradation/activated formation of ECM and/or (b) attenuated migration/mobilisation of granulocytes and/or (c) direct effect on Lindan and its interactions with the ECM and/or (d) reduced susceptibility of HSC against Lindan. Further studies are needed to distinguish between these possibilities, but a multiple targeting approach seems to be the most likely explanation for the documented findings.

PG5-07

Transmission of ultraviolet light in potentized substances and controls

Wolf U[1,2], Wolf M[1,2], Heusser P[1], Thurneysen A[1], Baumgartner S[1,2]

[1]Institute of Complementary Medicine KIKOM, University of Berne, Switzerland; [2]National High Magnetic Field Laboratory, Tallahassee, USA

Background: Many clinical trials show a significant effect of potentized substances. This effectiveness is difficult to explain within a conventional scientific context, particularly when dilutions beyond Avogadro's number are employed. Therefore, it is important to study, whether potentized substances have specific physical properties, which could lead to an understanding of their mode of action and thus provide a scientific basis for their use in medicine. **Objective:** We studied the transmission of UV-light in potentized quartz (SiO2), sulfur (S) and copper sulfate (CuSO4). Since our preliminary measurements had shown a lower transmission of UV-light for CuSO4 we intended to verify these findings and to also investigate other substances using a rigorous protocol. **Material and Methods:** Potentized dilutions of SiO2 (centesimal, c), S (decimal, x) and CuSO4 (centesimal, c) and controls (successed potentization medium) were prepared in a high class clean room, randomized and blinded. UV-measurements were performed with a Perkin-Elmer Lambda IIIB spectrometer and each sample and control was measured 5 times. Transmission (in %) from 215 to 290nm and across the five measurements was averaged and the mean values and standard deviations for potencies and controls were determined. Inorganic trace analysis of all samples was effectuated by inductively coupled plasma mass-spectrometry (ICP-MS). **Results:** The mean differences in transmission ± SE (%) between potentized substances and controls and the significances were: CuSO4 : -0.0351 ± 0.0136% , p= 0.0124. SiO2 : -0.0323 ± 0.0205% , p= 0.0630. S : -0.0281 ± 0.0409% , p= 0.5321. The transmission in all potentized substances was by 0.0318±0.0035% smaller than in the controls and the variability was larger by a factor 1.39±0.25 (not significant: F-test). Contamination, measured by ICP-MS, was negligible (<10 ppb) for all ions. **Conclusion:** Potentized CuSO4 has a significantly lower transmission compared to controls. The effect size, i.e. the difference in transmission is remarkably similar for all three substances. The higher variability for the potencies may indicate that transmission at the different dilution levels constitutes a pattern with peaks and troughs as described by L. Kolisko.

PG5-08

Homeopathic treatment in cancer patients – a retrospective data analysis

Guethlin C[1], Hinrichs I[1], Walach H[2], Rostock M[3]

[1]Department of Evaluation Research in Complementary Medicine, University Medical Center Freiburg, Germany; [2]School of Social Sciences, University of Northampton, UK; [3]Tumor Biology Center at Albert Ludwigs University Freiburg, Germany

Aims: To inform a prospective pilot study comparing homeopathy with conventional treatment in cancer patients it was considered necessary to look into already available retrospective data on homeopathy in cancer patients. We choose a very detailed and complex retrospective study design outlined here together with some results. **Methods:** The data analysis consisted of a best case analysis and a randomized study part. In the best case analysis data files of those patients were analysed who clearly benefited from homeopathy according to the homeopath. In the second study part data files were randomly drawn from the filing system of a special homeopathic in- and outpatient clinic. Both parts together included 123 patients; the outcomes were evaluated by the homeopath and by an independent oncological expert and by the patients themselves. **Results:** Both study groups were astonishingly equivalent in their patient characteristics: 65% were female, most of them had breast cancer. 71 % had had an appropriate conventional therapy in their past. 55% used homeopathy in a complementary approach, 17% used it alternatively and 28% reduced the conventional therapy due to homeopathy. The patients and the homeopaths rated homeopathy as being beneficial with respect to quality of life and some cancer response. Whereas homeopaths also assumed longer survival times for their best cases due to the homeopathic treatment this impression could not be clearly and reliable vindicated by the oncological expert. **Conclusion:** Homeopathy is considered to be beneficial by patients and homeopaths with respect to quality of life and cancer issues. However, the only way to study survival is by a prospective study design, which was proposed in a second study, together with this retrospective analysis (second study not yet finished).

PG5-09

Do glass-derived silicates induce neuroprotective effects observed following intravenously administered serially-diluted glutamate: A putative mechanism for 'homeopathic' effects

Ives J[1], Moffett J[2], Arun P[2], Hartings J[3], Olufade A[3], Williams A[3], Tortella F[3], Todorov T[4], Centeno J[4], Somiari R[5], Namboodiri A[2], Jonas W[1]

[1]Samueli Institute for Information Biology, Alexandria, USA; [2]Departments of Anatomy, Physiology and Genetics, Uniformed Services University of the Health Sciences, Bethesda, USA; [3]Department of Neuropharmacology and Molecular Biology, Walter Reed Army Institute of Research, Silver Spring, USA; [4]Armed Forces Institute of Pathology, Washington, USA; [5]Windber Research Institute, Windber, USA

We report here that homeopathically prepared glutamate significantly decreased infarct size and significantly improved neurological scores in rats subjected to 2 hours of transient middle cerebral artery occlusion (MCAo) as compared with control solutions. Trace element analyses of the experimental and control solutions indicated that they contained micromolar concentrations of silicon, sodium, and boron, which were found to be derived from the borosilicate glass vials used to generate the homeopathic preparations. The levels of silicon in the experimental solutions were found to be nearly double those of the control solutions stored in glass vials, whereas the concentrations of the other solutes were similar. To further investigate this neuroprotective affect, uninjured rats were administered the same experimental and control solutions used for the MCAo study according to the same schedule. Striatal tissue was isolated, homogenized, and subjected to high-throughput 2D-DIGE proteomics followed by mass spectroscopy of the proteins with altered expression. Thirty protein spots were expressed at different levels (28 upregulated) in the striatum of the experimental animals. The altered proteins were associated with oxidative-stress responses, regulation of protein synthesis, vesicle trafficking, and energy metabolism. We hypothesize that silicates derived from glass vials may be responsible for certain actions of homeopathic preparations, including the neuroprotective effects observed here.

Acknowledgements: Research was supported by the Samueli Institute for Information Biology (G170-ON), NIH grant R21AT00178, and DoD funding.

PG5-10

Efficacy, long-term efficiency and cost-effectiveness of homeopathy in inattentive children

von Ammon K[1], Frei H[2], Thurneysen A[1]

[1]Institute of Complementary Medicine KIKOM, University of Berne, Switzerland; [2]Swiss Association of Homeopathic Physicians SAHP, Laupen BE, Switzerland

Introduction: ADHD recently has reached a prevalence of 3-5% in school children. In Switzerland, stimulant prescriptions increased sevenfold between 1992 and 1999. Parents, physicians and psychologists were looking for other treatment options. Two clinical studies suggested homeopathy to be effective in ADHD children. **Objective:** To demonstrate suitability, efficacy, clinical and cost effectiveness in children with attention deficit disorder with/without hyperactivity (ADHD/ADD). **Method:** Notice of clinical, behavioural and cognitive improvements in affected children during homeopathic treatment induced a prospective, observational pilot study to gain statistic data. Next steps were the design of a randomised clinical trial (RCT) with a combination of conventional, classical homeopathic and long-term follow-up requirements, approval of the ethics committee and collecting funds. A double blind placebo controlled crossover RCT included in a prospective observational study was conducted uneventfully. **Results:** Elaborated classical homeopathy proved (i) clinical efficiency and particular neuropsychological improvement ($p<.0001$), stable for more than 5 years follow-up, (ii) efficacy of the remedies ($p<.05$), and (iii) economic comparison with stimulants to be in favor for homeopathy with increasing treatment duration and stimulant doses. Adaptations of diagnostic, therapeutic, data processing and analytic procedures had been implemented to improve effectiveness and enabling a detailed evaluation. **Discussion:** The results point at a specific action of homeopathic remedies despite the unknown mechanism of action, to long-term stability of efficiency and cost-effectiveness of classical homeopathic therapy in children with ADD/ADHD. **Conclusion:** Long-term strategy enabled development, implementation, realisation and successful conclusion of a new study design combining economic and both, conventional and homeopathic, demands.

PG5-11

Is a unified theory of homeopathy and conventional medicine possible?

Milgrom LR

Imperial College London, UK

Background: Greater integration of CAMs with conventional health provision is being called for, but will CAMs be mere 'add-ons', with homeopathy providing controversy, or could richer, more complex relationships exist between homeopathy and conventional medicine? Finding possible theoretical links between these two contradictory disciplines might be of interest. Thus homeopathy uses the ancient concept of a self-regulating Vital Force (Vf). Disturbance of the Vf is thought to result in dis-ease manifestation (observed as multi-levelled symptom expression), as it attempts to restore holistic balance. Treatment attempts to aid the Vf in its struggle. Conventional medicine (allopathy) on the other hand, takes a deterministic view of disease: external agents (viruses, bacteria, etc) or internal biochemical imbalances (e.g., genetic abnormalities), are considered causes of pathology. Treatment is geared towards eradicating these causative disease factors, sometimes at the expense of the homeostatic immune system. A mathematical metaphor describing the Vf as a 'quantised gyroscope', equates strength of symptom expression to degree of Vf 'gyroscopic' precession: complete removal of symptoms corresponds to cessation of 'precession'. This approach interprets diseases and homeopathic remedies respectively as braking and accelerating 'torques' on Vf 'angular momentum'. **Method:** Approximations applied to the Vf 'wave function' provide possible insights into why conventional medicine so readily dismisses the action of highly potentised homeopathic remedies. In addition, a simple geometric force diagram provides another mathematical metaphor this time to begin modelling allopathic drug action and immune system reaction. **Results:** The two mathematical metaphors converge on the same result: that from a conventional medical perspective, homeopathic remedies potentised beyond Avogadro's number should exert no clinically observable effects. **Conclusion:** By following the logic of the mathematical metaphors presented in this paper, it is suggested that eventually conventional medicine might come to be seen as a special case of a broader therapeutic paradigm. The implications for the possible integration of conventional medicine with homeopathy are discussed.

PG6-01

An organic diet can increase the levels of conjugated linoleic acids in the breast milk of lactating women

Simões-Wüst AP[1], Rist L[1], Mueller A[2], Barthel C[2], Snijders B[3], Jansen M[4], Huber M[5], Kummeling I[3], von Mandach U[6], Steinhart H[2], Thijs C[3]

[1]Research Department, Paracelsus Hospital Richterswil, Switzerland; [2]Institute of Biochemistry and Food Chemistry, Department of Food Chemistry, University of Hamburg, Germany; [3]Department of Epidemiology, Nutrition and Toxicology Research Institute Maastricht (Nutrim) and Care and Public Health Research Institute (Caphri), Maastricht University, The Netherlands; [4]TNO Nutrition and Food Research, Zeist, The Netherlands; [5]Louis Bolk Institute, Driebergen, The Netherlands; [6]Department of Obstetrics, Zurich University Hospital, Switzerland

Background: Organic food is being demanded by a growing group of consumers that perceive it as healthier and a few life style studies suggest that this food could attenuate the development of allergic/atopic diseases. At the molecular level, the favourable effects of conjugated linoleic acid isomers (CLA) on human health are currently receiving attention in nutritional research. Among others, immune-modulating effects of CLA have been described. Our aim was to find out whether the incorporation of organic dairy and meat products in the maternal diet affects the contents of CLA and *trans*-vaccenic acid (TVA, a CLA precursor) in human breast milk. **Methods:** To this purpose, milk samples from 312 breastfeeding mothers participating in the KOALA Birth Cohort Study were collected 1 month postpartum and analysed for fatty acid composition. The participants had documented varying lifestyles in relation to the use of conventional or organic products. **Results:** The content of the most common CLA, rumenic acid (RA) increased in a statistically significant way while going from a conventional diet (no organic dairy/meat products, 0.25 wt%, n=186) to a moderately organic diet (50–90% organic dairy/meat, 0.29 wt%, n=33, p=0.02) and to a strict organic diet (>90% organic dairy/meat, 0.34 wt%, n=37, p≤0.001). The levels of TVA were augmented among the participants with a moderately organic diet (0.54 wt%) and those with a strict organic diet (0.59 wt%, p≤0.001), in comparison with the conventional group (0.48 wt%). After adjusting for covariables (recruitment group, maternal age, maternal education, use of supplements and season), statistical significance was retained in the group of strict organic dairy users (p<0.001 for RA). **Conclusion:** Levels of RA and TVA in human milk can be modulated if breast-feeding mothers replace conventional dairy and/or meat products by organic ones. Interestingly, it has been shown that the levels of CLA in cow's milk from organic producers in Europe are significantly higher as CLA levels in the milk from conventional producers. Therefore, and since the fat from human breast milk is likely to be of dietary origin, we believe that the larger amounts of RA and TVA in breast milk from the organic groups were due to the corresponding intake of organic dairy and meat products. A potential contribution of CLA to health-improvement will be briefly discussed.

PG6-02

Results of a modified Delphi consensus-building process to classify natural and physical healing methods in relation to "Traditional European Medicine (TEM)"

Uehleke B

Department of Natural Medicine, Charite University Medicine Berlin, Germany

Aims: To identify which methods of natural medicine and CAM are to be regarded as part of "Traditional European Medicine (TEM)". In the second step a proposal for a definition of TEM is discussed briefly as a basis for a further consensus-finding process. **Methods:** Two questionnaires with two-time evaluation, anonymous except to the facilitator, were sent to an expert panel comprising 19 academic experts on naturopathy and 5 experts on medical history of naturopathy. The first questionnaire contained 20 questions including control questions about the characteristics and relations of alternative healing methods to naturopathy or TEM, which were to be answered with either "yes", "no" or "depending on .."; in case of the latter participants were asked to provide a free-text argument. The second step consisted of a proposal for a definition, contents and arguments for TEM to be evaluated by means of ratings and free text. **Results:** 15 experts on naturopathy and 4 experts on medical history completed the first questionnaire. A clear majority suggest that TEM should be developed and defined as a defined medicinal system with its own history-based philosophy. It was stressed by several experts that TEM should have a better relation to its historical basis than "Traditional Chinese Medicine" does. A broad majority regards balneotherapy, hydrotherapy, nutritional therapy, physical exercise, massage techniques, and herbal medicine as parts of TEM, whereas homeopathy and electrotherapy would not belong to TEM. The numerous individual comments on the proposed definition and characteristics of TEM found in the second part give reason to continue with the consensus-finding process by organising at least one more meeting, thereby allowing intensive discussion to take place. **Conclusions:** There is a sufficient majority among experts to justify a further systematic development of the term "TEM", with the aim of establishing a more precise medical system than that vaguely characterized by "naturopathy".

PG6-03

Use of an elder-based herbal hypocaloric diet as a starter for lifestyle change

Chrubasik C[1], Wiesner L[1], Torda T[2], Chrubasik S[1]

[1]Department of Forensic Medicine, University of Freiburg, Germany;
[2]School of Medical Sciences, University of New South Wales, Sydney, Australia

Aim: Aim of the study was, to investigate an elder-based herbal hypocaloric diet as a start to lifestyle change in persons who considered themselves overweight. **Methods:** With consent of the Human Ethics Committee of the University of Freiburg, 90 consecutive participants who wished to loose weight were included. Pregnant women, diabetics, epileptics and people with severe organic diseases were excluded. After initial assessments for weight, well-being and quality of life on 10-point numeric rating scales, participants were instructed to measure their blood pressure (BP, Boso-medicus PC®) and received the diet kindly provided by Dr. Dünner GmbH, Switzerland: 2–3 teaspoons of psyllium in the mornings for 2 weeks with sufficient liquid. On days 5–12 meal replacements by elderberry (EB) juice (200 ml EB concentrate/day supplemented with elderflower (EF) juice and extract, diluted 1:5, yielding 400 kcal/d – total liquid intake not less than 3 l/day) and a total of 225 mg dried EB powder, 600 mg EF extract (as a mixture) and 2.7 g asparagus powder daily in tablet form. BP measurements on days 1–4 were averaged for pre-treatment values. From days 9 to 14, BP was recorded again. Participants received a diary, to document any food intake and occurrence of adverse events (AE) and, were recommended to make plans for a change in lifestyle after the diet. On the final visit, weight, well-being and quality of life were again assessed. **Results:** Ten participants dropped out (6 before beginning the diet, 3 discontinued due to AE (in 2, related to the diet), 1 failed to attend the final visit). Of the 80 completers (ITT population: 34 men, 36 women), 23 admitted to have broken the diet. Weight had decreased by 3.2 ± 1.9 kg (mean±SD, p< 0.001), BMI from 29.9 ± 5.2 to 28.9 ± 5.0 kg/m2 (p<0.001), systolic BP from 129±13 to 122±13 mmHg (p<0.001) and diastolic BP from 80±9 to 78±9 mm Hg (p<0.001). In hypertensive participants, the fall in systolic BP correlated with weight loss (p=0.047). Physical and emotional well-being, had improved significantly (all p<0.001), likewise the quality of life (p<0.01). 57 patients (including the drop-outs) reported a total of 79 AEs; none was severe. **Conclsuion:** Most patients benefited from the elder-based hypocaloric diet in terms of weight loss, blood pressure decrease and increased well-being and quality of life. However, it is known that only continuous lifestyle changes will result in long-term success.

PG6-04

Marine omega-3 fatty acids intake among Quebecers (Canada): Where are we compared to worldwide recommendations?

Dodin S, Lucas M, Asselin G, Plourde M, Cunnane SC, Dewailly E

Lucie et André Chagnon Chair's for the teaching of an integrated approach in prevention, Laval University, Saint-François d'Assise Hospital (CHUQ), Québec (QC) Canada

Background: Marine omega-3 (n-3) fatty acids intake, eicosapentaenoic (EPA) and docosahexaenoic acids (DHA), have been associated with beneficial effects in health. Although n-3 have gained in popularity during last years, little is known about actual marine n-3 intake of Quebecers. **Methods:** We quantified marine products and marine n-3 intake among a representative sample (n=1001) of adults from the province of Quebec. EPA and DHA intake were estimated from a FFQ on marine products completed by participants in a telephone survey and compared with the worldwide recommendations. Mean (±SD) and median EPA+DHA intakes for all participants were respectively estimated at 305±329 mg/d and 216 mg/d. **Results:** Proportion of Quebecers who had an intake lower than the international recommendation for prevention of cardiovascular diseases (500 mg EPA+DHA/d) was 82.4% (CI 95%: 79.9–84.9). Mean (±SD) and median DHA intakes among childbearing-aged women (n=120, 18–34 yrs) were respectively estimated at 182±17 mg/d and 136 mg/d. Proportion of childbearing women who had adequate intake of DHA as recommended by the Perinatal Lipid Nutrition (PERILIP) (>200 mg DHA/d) and the International Society for the Study of Fatty Acids and Lipids (ISSFAL) (>300 mg DHA/d) were respectively of 30% and 17%. Thirteen percent of Quebecers take more than one capsule of marine n-3 or fish oil per day. **Conclsuion:** Marine products and n-3 consumption among Quebecers appear to be lower than international recommendations. Since marine n-3 consumption confers health benefits and may reduce health costs, strategies aiming to increase their consumption should be implemented to improve public health in Quebecers (Canada).

PG6-05

RCT in breast cancer patients affected by severe chronic tumour-associated fatigue

Kennemann C, Lüdtke R, Franken U, Paul A, Dobos G, Spahn G

Chair of Complementary Medicine, University of Duisburg-Essen; Department of Internal and Integrative Medicine, Kliniken Essen-Mitte, Germany

We conducted a randomised controlled intervention study in 55 breast cancer patients (aged 33–75) who showed high fatigue scores more than three months after active tumour treatment. 25 patients were allocated to a home-based pulse controlled walking group under the supervision of a sport instructor (duration 10 weeks, minimal 3 × 30 min of moderate walking exercise per week), 30 patients took part in a 10 weeks multimodal mind-body programme including moderate walking exercise, hydrotherapy, nutrition, relaxation, stress reduction, cognitive restructuring and an introduction to techniques of mindfulness (MBSR) by a multiprofessional team. Fatigue, anxiety and depression, life quality and functional well-being were assessed with standard questionnaires for oncology patients (MFI-20, FAQ subscales, EORTC-QLQ C30, Menopausal rating scale, HADS) at the entry and the end of the study and also three months post-intervention. Fatigue in a homogeneous study population of breast cancer patients suffering of chronic fatigue was markedly reduced in both the control group (exercise only) and the multimodal intervention group without significant differences between the two groups. Marked improvement was also seen in parameters of life quality and general functional well-being. Fatigue patients who suffered of pain or anxiety showed a better outcome after the multimodal intervention with significantly reduced scores in these symptoms compared to the control group.

PG6-06

Structuring and evaluation of an obligatory credited course in '*rehabilitation, physical therapy and naturopathy*' at the University of Duisburg-Essen, Germany

Roy N, Klose P, Heue M, Dobos GJ

Chair of Complementary Medicine, University of Duisburg-Essen; Department of Internal and Integrative Medicine, Kliniken Essen-Mitte, Germany

Aim: This work presents a model of integrating domain 12 – academics, especially naturopathy, into the curriculum of conventional western medicine at German universities. Starting in winter term 2005/2006, all universities in Germany providing education in Medicine were committed to develop a contemporary curriculum for prospective medical practitioners, including scientifically verified and evidence-based naturopathy as well as conventional medicine. In addition to selecting the major topics and their presentation, it was necessary to assure the quality of didactics by an evaluation process. **Methods:** The medical association questionnaire for advanced training of medical practitioners was utilized. Further, the student's comments on each single questionnaire were collected and analyzed according to the categories of an established gauge for educational evaluations of the University of Linz, Austria, in accordance with the official teaching-evaluation of the University of Duisburg-Essen, which is also based on these categories. **Results**: There were no differences of students' acceptance comparing the voluntarily visited lectures with the obligatory seminars. As a result, both weak points of the own evaluation could be found and the development of optimised inquiry was possible (concerning organization of all activities and social quality, conditions, mood during lecture or seminar). Furthermore, the idea of combining the electronic evaluation of the university and the internal questionnaire in direct comparison came up and was implemented. **Discussion:** The concept presents a model of integrating "*rehabilitation, physical therapy and naturopathy*" at national and international universities. It fulfills the criteria of the Medical Association´s professional code of conduct (national) and fosters a change of medical education which is now aimed more explicitly at patient's needs and satisfaction. Furthermore, the course was enthusiastically accepted by students, since it fulfils their need of a practical and patient-oriented medical education.

PG7-01

Spirituality/religiosity, life satisfaction and disease perception in patients with chronic pain diseases

Büssing A[1], Balzat HJ[2], Ostermann T[1]

[1]Department of Medical Theory and Complementary Medicine, Faculty of Medicine, University of Witten/Herdecke, Germany; [2]Pain Out-Patient Clinic, Gemeinschaftskrankenhaus Herdecke, Germany

Aim: We intended to analyse spirituality and religiosity (SpR) and their impact on dealing with illness in patients with chronic pain diseases. **Methods:** We enrolled 154 patients (54±13 y, f:m=4.0; 57% married; 53% secondary school, 19% junior high school, 14% high school; 88% Christian affiliation) which were treated at a pain outpatient clinic. All were assured of confidentiality, gave informed consent, and completed the questionnaires by themselves, i.e. SpREUK, AKU-Pain, Disease Interpretation according to Lipowski, Huebner´s Brief Multidimensional Life Satisfaction Scale. **Results:** Among the adaptive coping styles, Search for external help (82±14) and Positivism & Fighting (75±14) had the highest relevance, followed by Chance & Meaning (68±20) and Trust in God´s help (62±32), which had the strongest variance. Patients did find Support in relations of life through SpR (SLSpR: 61±29) and had Trust in higher source (THS: 58±32). Search for meaningful support raised low interest (SMS: 42±29), while Positive interpretation of disease had intermediate levels (PID: 51±24). SLSpR significantly correlated with life satisfaction aspects (self: r=0.359; future prospects: r=0.381), and THS with life satisfaction (self: r=0.235; future prospects: r=0.223). The aspects family life, friends, work, living area or financial situation did not correlate with SpR. 67% perceived their pain disease as an interrupt/loss. Perception of disease as a Value strongly correlated with SMS (r=0.527), PID (r=0.567), THS (r=0.373) and SLSpR (r=0.375); perception as Challenge correlated with all 4 SpREUK scales (SMS: r=0.492), THS (r=0.449), PID (r=0.497), and SLSpR (r=0.328). Disease perception as a Cry for help correlated with SMS (r=0.355) and PID (r=0.331). None of the SpREUK scales correlated with disease perception as Enemy, Punishment or Weakness. **Conclusion:** Several patients regard SpR as helpful. Moreover, aspects of life satisfaction and positive disease perception are connected with SpR issues. Because 44% would like to talk with their medical doctor about their SpR needs, and only 26% with a priest, these issues should be carefully addressed in the care for patients with chronic disease.

PG7-02

Mindfulness based coping with university life – implementing and evaluating a new intervention

Lynch SM[1], Walach H[1,2]

[1]School of Psychology, University of Northampton, UK; [2]Samueli Institute, European Office, Northampton, UK

Aims: University life is accompanied by an array of potential stressors such as changing relationships, new living environments and the pressure to get good grades (Furr et al., 2001). The mental health of students appears to be declining (Royal College of Psychiatrists, 2003) and while the forces behind this decline are not clear, what is clear is that appropriate psychosocial support should be available to help students navigate the often turbulent waters of university life. The goal of this study is to develop and pilot test an 8 week group psychosocial intervention of mindfulness-based coping with university life (MBCUL), tailored to the specific needs of students, both in terms of content and structure, based on the highly successful mindfulness-based stress reduction (MBSR) programme developed by Jon Kabat-Zinn. **Method:** A pre test/post test mixed methods research design will be employed. Participants' mood (HADS), level of mindfulness (Freiburg mindfulness inventory) and individualised goals, will be measured both before and after attending the MBCUL programme. Qualitative interviews will be conducted to gain an understanding of both students' expectations and experience of the programme. The study will be conducted at the University of Northampton and will consist of 1, or given enough interest, 2 groups of 8-15 university undergraduates recruited from campus advertising. Participants will have an initial interview and complete the Time 1 quantitative measures prior to the course commencement. At Time 2, after the 8 week MBCUL programme, participants will be interviewed again and complete the second set of quantitative measures. The qualitative interviews will be analysed using appropriate techniques. **Results:** First results will be available for presentation. If the results suggest the MBCUL programme is effective in improving mood and mindfulness and is reported as beneficial by participants, it will form the basis of a larger scale randomised study examining the physiological, psychological, cognitive and social impact of attending MBCUL. **Conclusion:** The potential benefits of a programme such as MBCUL are obvious. While not changing the issues faced, it would provide students with an effective means of coping with such issues, the benefits of which may be felt well beyond graduation.

PG7-03

Disturbed neuroendocrine-immune communication as a link to Mind/Body Medicine in inflammatory bowel diseases (IBD)

Langhorst J, Elsenbruch S, Cobelens P, Lucas A, Benson S, Kavelaars A, Heijnen CJ, Schedlowski M, Dobos GJ

Chair of Complementary and Integrative Medicine, University of Duisburg-Essen, Department of Internal Medicine, Kliniken Essen-Mitte, Germany

Background: Mind/Body interactions, like psychological stress, and depressive symptoms have been found to play a role in disease initiation and exacerbation in inflammatory bowel diseases (IBD; Ulcerative Colitis: UC; Crohn´s Disease: CD). However, the mechanisms remain unclear. The goal in our study was to address neuroendocrine-immune interactions in patients with IBD. **Methods:** IBD patients and healthy controls were recruited for two experiments: 1) In an in vitro stress model the effects of the b-adrenergic agonist terbutaline and the glucocorticoid agonist dexamethasone on LPS-stimulated TNF-a and IL-10 production in peripheral blood cells were investigated in N=46 IBD pts (N=32 in remission and N=14 with active disease) with a perceived impact of subjective distress and N=19 controls. 2) Neuroendocrine and cellular immune responses to a standard laboratory stressor (public speaking) were compared in N=23 with UC in remission and N=25 controls, including the analysis of the redistribution of circulating lymphocytes and of the production of LPS-stimulated TNF-a and IL-10, and of CD2/CD28-stimulated IL-10 and IFN-g. **Results:** 1) Whereas controls showed a significant and concentration-dependent increase in IL-10 production in response to terbutaline, this response was significantly diminished in IBD in remission as well as in active disease (ANOVA group effects: both p<.01). Interestingly, this reduction in IL-10 response to terbutaline was more pronounced in active IBD compared to IBD in remission (ANOVA group effects: both p<.05). At the same time, concentration-dependent suppression of TNF- a production by both terbutaline and dexamethasone was comparable in IBD and controls. 2) The stress-induced redistribution of circulating leukocytes and lymphocyte subpopulations were comparable in IBD and controls. Significant stress-induced increases in TNF-a, IL-10 and IFN-g were observed in both groups (all ANOVA time effects: p<.01), with no difference between the groups. **Conclusions:** These data provide further evidence that adrenergic-immune interactions are disturbed in IBD, irrespective of the diagnosis. Given the pivotal role of pro-and anti-inflammatory cytokines in IBD pathophysiology, our findings of disturbed adrenergic IL-10 regulation in the in vitro stress model, which was particularly pronounced during disease exacerbation, could be part of the mechanism(s) underlying the modulation of disease activity by psychological stress. These findings support a further integration of Mind/Body Medicine techniques in the treatment of IBD.

PG7-04

Mindfulness based stress reduction in patients with fibromyalgia – a randomized controlled trial

Jena S, Schmidt S, Grossman P, Schwarzer B, Naumann J, Walach H

Department of Evaluation Research in Complementary Medicine, Institute for Environmental Medicine, University Medical Centre Freiburg, Germany

Aims: Mindfulness-based stress reduction (MBSR), an eight week group program, has been shown to produce health benefits in a number of pilot studies, uncontrolled observational studies, and randomized investigations of chronic pain disorders. Fibromyalgia is a clinical syndrome with chronic pain, fatigue, and sleep disorders as major symptoms. The effectiveness of an eight week mindfulness based group program (MBSR) on fibromyalgia patients was investigated. **Method:** Because fibromyalgia is almost exclusively a female disorder, we have limited this study to women. In a three arm randomized controlled trial 176 female patients were randomized to either (i) a waiting list (ii) an active control to account for nonspecific effects of treatment or (iii) MBSR. The main outcome criteria are self-reported and fibromyalgia-specific quality of life as well as general quality of life at 4 month post treatment. In addition a Biobehavioral Fibromyalgia Index composed of a variety of psychophysiological and behavioral variables will be computed. This index will be generated from data gathered via an ambulatory psychophysiological monitoring system, which comprises parameters of mobility, sleep quality, and cardiovascular well-being. Primary and secondary outcome variables (depression score, pain quality, anxiety, mindfulness, compliance, number of tender points, other therapeutic measures) were assessed at beginning and end of the training, as well as at 4- and 12-month post-treatment. **Results:** At baseline patients had an average tender point pain count of 15.3 (out of 18) and an average age of 54 years. 31.8% completed the German equivalent of the A-level (13 years in school). None of the baseline characteristics showed significant differences between the groups. Overall 138 patients (79%) completed the study. Primary outcome measures are compared for the three interventions at post-intervention and at 4 months and 12 months follow-up. Data evaluation is ongoing and will be finished by February. **Conclusion:** On the basis of this trial it will be possible to decide whether MBSR has beneficial effects for patients with fibromyalgia and whether these effects, should they be present, are due to the specific effects of mindfulness or rather non-specific.

PG7-05

Healing the heart: A randomized pilot study of a spiritual retreat for acute coronary syndrome patients

Warber SL, Ingerman S, Wunder J, Schreiber A, Gillespie BW, Durda K, Moura VL, Smith K, Rhodes K, Rubenfire M

University of Michigan Integrative Medicine, Ann Arbor, USA

Aims: In ischemic heart disease, depression is associated with increased risk of cardiovascular morbidity and mortality. Spirituality is associated with less depression and improved cardiac outcomes, however, few interventions to enhance spirituality have been tested. We studied the effects of a non-denominational spiritual retreat, Medicine for the Earth (MFTE), versus a lifestyle change program (LCP) or usual cardiac care in persons recovering from acute coronary syndrome (ACS). Outcomes of interest were depression, spiritual well-being, perceived stress, and hope. **Methods:** Recent ACS patients (n=58) were recruited via local and national (USA) advertising. After randomization, 11 declined; 40 completed the study. At the 4-day MFTE retreat, participants learned to transcend ego, connect with divinity, and heal each other spiritually using guided imagery, meditation, drumming, journal writing, and nature-based ritual. At the 4-day LCP retreat, participants learned nutrition, exercise, and stress management. Retreat participants received bi-weekly phone coaching for 3 months. The third group received usual cardiac care throughout. Validated self-report scales were collected at baseline, immediately post retreat, and 3 and 6 months later. Data were evaluated using repeated measures linear models. **Results:** Both intervention groups shifted from mild-moderate depression at baseline into the normal range immediately after the retreats and at 3 and 6 months. However, the time trends between groups were not significantly different (p=0.21). The 'reflective' subscale of spiritual well-being was significantly improved over time by being at the MFTE retreat (p=0.015), while 'wholeness' significantly improved over time across all groups (p=0.02). Perceived stress was reduced by both retreats, but the LCP group had a rise in perceived stress at 3 months (p=0.049). Hope was markedly improved by the MFTE retreat, an effect that persisted for 3 and 6 months following the intervention (p=0.014). **Conclusions:** This pilot study shows that a spiritual retreat, MFTE, increases hope while reducing depression and perceived stress in persons with ACS. We conclude that MFTE is worthy of a larger trial.

PG7-06

Efficacy of a mind-body intervention for patients with terminal diseases and their caregivers

Vincent A, Cha S, Kaur JS, Bauer BA, Wahner-Roedler DL

Mayo Clinic, Rochester, USA

Aims: To evaluate the efficacy of a mind-body intervention on Quality of Life (QOL) of patients with terminal diseases and their caregivers. Tertiary medical centers in the USA are often the place where patients learn about a terminal diagnoses. To help patients and their caregivers cope with the experience of loss, grieving, support from personnel trained in mind-body interventions is a logical approach. **Methods:** Patients: 29 patients and their care givers with incurable diseases identified by the Complementary and Integrative Medicine Service were enrolled in the study. Personnel: A Complementary and Integrative Medicine practitioner trained in shamanic medicine delivered the intervention in two visits. Intervention: Visit 1: The interview was started with the question" What are you feeling within yourself?" The patients and caregivers were then given a questionnaire to be reviewed prior to the next visit which included questions regarding their fears, unfinished and unresolved issues, meaning of the disease, and meaning of healing. Visit 2: During this visit, the patient and caregiver discussed the contents of the questionnaire with the practitioner acting as a listener. The goal was to enable patients and caregivers to attain peace in their own mind and a sense of wholeness and completion. The patient was encouraged to share their joys and blessings with the practitioner, family and friends. Instrument: a validated LASA form on QOL regarding physical, emotional, spiritual, intellectual and overall well-being was administered to patients and care givers on the first visit and 2-3 days post intervention. Statistics: Analysis was performed using matched pair method for differences pre and post intervention. **Results:** Statistically significant improvement was seen in patients' physical (p=0.0007), emotional (p<0.0054), spiritual (p=0.0251) and overall well-being (p=0.0037). Statistically significant improvement was also seen in caregivers' physical (p=0.0002), emotional (p<0.0001), and overall well-being (p< 0.0001). No significant changes were seen in the caregivers' spiritual well being or the patients' or caregivers' intellectual well-being. **Conclusion:** A mind-body intervention utilizing a reflective questionnaire and a reflective session mediated by an individual trained in shamanic medicine improves several aspects of QOL for patients with terminal diseases and their caregivers.

PG7-07

A pilot study of yoga treatment for menopausal symptoms

Booth-LaForce C[1], Taylor MR[1], Thurston RC[2], Elven EC[1]

[1]School of Nursing, University of Washington, USA; [2]Department of Psychiatry, University of Pittsburgh, USA

Aims: To assess the feasibility and efficacy of a yoga treatment for menopausal symptoms. Both physiologic and self-reported measures of hot flashes were included. **Methods:** A prospective within-group pilot study was conducted in the U.S. Participants were 12 peri- and post-menopausal women with at least 4 menopausal hot flashes per day, at least 4 days per week. Assessments were administered before and after completion of a 10-week community-based yoga program. Pre- and post-treatment measures included: Severity of questionnaire-rated menopausal symptoms (Wiklund Symptom Check List), number and intensity of hot flashes (24-hr ambulatory skin-conductance monitoring; hot-flash diary), interference of hot flashes with daily life (Hot Flash Related Daily Interference), and subjective sleep quality (Pittsburgh Sleep Quality Index). Yoga classes included breathing techniques, postures, and relaxation poses designed specifically for menopausal symptoms. Participants were asked to practice at home 15 minutes each day in addition to weekly classes. Post-treatment interviews were conducted to gauge the women's reactions to the study and their perceptions of yoga effects. T-tests for paired samples were used to evaluate changes from pre- to post-treatment. **Results:** Eleven women completed the study and attended a mean of 7.45 (SD 1.63) classes. The following changes occurred from pre- to post-treatment: Decreased severity of questionnaire-rated total menopausal symptoms (p=.04), decreased hot-flash daily interference (p=.05), and improved sleep efficiency (p=.02) and quality (p=.009). Neither 24-hr monitoring nor accompanying diaries yielded significant changes in hot flashes. Responses to post-treatment interview questions indicated an overall positive reaction to the study assessment procedures and to the yoga classes. The women reported positive changes in their hot flashes, night sweats, fatigue, anxiety, and irritability. Other effects of yoga for them included feeling physically good, more relaxed/calm, more flexible, stronger, better able to handle stress, more self-aware, and more energetic. **Conclusions:** The yoga treatment and study procedures were feasible for midlife women. Improvement in symptom perceptions and well-being warrant further study of yoga for menopausal symptoms, with a larger number of women and including a control group.

PG7-08

Subjective effects of deep field relaxation, a form of spiritual healing, on cancer patients – a qualitative study

Walach H, Schwarzer T, Boencke A, Müller S, Seiter C, Weis J

University of Northampton, School of Social Sciences & Samueli Institute European Office

Aims: Many cancer patients, especially in late stages, seek out alternative treatments, and often they use spiritual healing. We offered a certain kind of healing, Deep Field Relaxation, to cancer patients in end or late stages of their disease. We wanted to study the immediate and mid-term subjective effects and find out whether the treatment was worth further investigation. **Methods:** The therapy involves a deep form of relaxation by the therapist entering a quiet mental space on behalf of the patient. We conducted open interviews around predefined topics before, immediately after and a third time after 8 weeks and collected questionnaire (FACT-G), as well as medical data. Evaluation of interviews followed an inductive approach similar to a grounded theory model. **Results:** 18 patients were treated and interviewed. Data suggest that none of the patients reported any negative experiences. Positive experiences varied in intensity and longevity. While five patients who had considerable previous experience with meditation or relaxation techniques found the reatment relaxing and positive but without any lasting effects and two patients were too vague about their experiences, all other patients reported experiences of deep relaxation and positive feelings. Not all of them attributed these to the treatment itself. Patients experienced the relationship and the therapeutic situation positively without exception. Being and feeling accepted as they are, with their disease, allowed patients to accept themselves. This had personal impacts to varying degrees. **Conclusions:** Deep Field Relaxation is a viable and generally accepted treatment that deserves further study. It remains to be seen whether apart from those obvious subjective improvements any changes of projected medical prognoses will be traceable.

PG8-01

Parental beliefs and use of complementary and traditional remedies for children

Robinson N[1], Lorenc A[1], Blair M[2]

[1]Centre for Complementary Healthcare and Integrated Medicine (CCHIM), Faculty of Health and Human Sciences, Thames Valley University, London, UK; [2]River Island Paediatric and Child Health Academic Centre, Imperial College, London, UK

Aims: To explore the role of parental beliefs in the use of complementary medicine (CM) for children; to identify the use of traditional remedies in a multi-ethnic child population. **Methods:** The 'Beliefs in Medicine' and 'Multidimensional Health Locus of Control' questionnaires were used in a parent-completed survey carried out in a multi-ethnic paediatric outpatient department in London. Details on use of and advice obtained on traditional remedies and over the counter complementary medicines and reasons for their use were captured. **Results:** 201 questionnaires were completed, 83% by the child's mother. A total of 37% of parents used CM for their child. Homeopathy and herbal medicine were most commonly used in particular. CM was most often used for infections, skin disorders and gastro-intestinal problems. Information on CM was obtained outside of the healthcare consultation (word of mouth/friends and family), 88% of CM was bought over the counter (average cost £9.66/treatment) and 54% of CM use was not reported to their doctor. Parents who used CM for their children had significantly stronger beliefs in the overuse of conventional medicine ($p=0.031$) and were more likely to use CM themselves ($p<0.001$). Regression analysis demonstrated that parental CM use and poor child health status were significant predictors of CM use ($p<0.001$ and $p<0.05$). **Conclusions:** CM is widely used in this child population and is often accessed outside of mainstream healthcare. Parents appear to be taking a self-management approach when using CM for their children. Parents' health beliefs and behaviour may affect their healthcare choices for their children, particularly as women are more likely to use CM, to consult the GP and are the main providers of childcare. It is important that parents, particularly mothers, are well informed on the safe use of CM for children.

PG8-02

A survey of users' perspectives and experiences of complementary and alternative medicine (CAM) in the management of fibromyalgia syndrome (FMS)

Hardy-Pickering RD[1], Adams N[1], Roe BH[1], Sim J[2]

[1]Faculty of Health and Applied Social Sciences, Liverpool John Moores University, UK; [2]Keele University, UK

Background and Aims: Fibromyalgia sufferers are documented as being high users of CAM, though there is currently limited extant literature regarding the effectiveness or efficacy of CAM interventions for FMS in order to provide justification for its provision within conventional medical services. This study explores the experiences and perspectives of members of FMS support groups in the UK regarding use and perceived benefits of using CAM therapies. **Methods:** A specifically devised anonymous self-completion postal questionnaire was utilised for the study and distributed to members and associates of the Fibromyalgia Association (FMA) UK (n=1300). University ethical approval was obtained. **Results:** A response rate of 63% was obtained. 82% of respondents reported usage of CAM as an adjuvant strategy to conventional NHS treatment. Most accessed CAM outside the NHS with 78% of respondents reporting beneficial effects. Most frequently accessed interventions were manipulation / massage) (35%), aromatherapy (30%) herbal medicine (30%) and meditation (28%), many respondents reported accessed several forms of CAM. 70% of respondents considered that NHS health professionals were not well informed about FMS and 52% considered they did not receive appropriate treatment from the NHS. No statistically significant relationships were found between variables. **Conclusions:** FMS sufferers perceive CAM therapies to be useful adjuvant interventions to conventional medical treatment which has implications for integration of CAM. The role of patient-practitioner relationships and provision of information were considered important components of the interventions and these aspects are being explored in ongoing research.

PG8-03

Patients with recent onset rheumatoid arthritis use complementary and alternative medicine irrespective of disease activity and kind of care

Westhoff G[1], Stange R[2], Zink A[1]

[1]Epidemiology Unit, German Rheumatism Research Centre, Berlin, Germany; [2]Department of Naturopathy Charité – University Berlin & Immanuel-Hospital Berlin, Germany

Objective: To investigate how many patients with recent onset rheumatoid arthritis (RA) use CAM and whether CAM is used alternatively or in addition to disease modifying antirheumatic drugs (DMARD). **Patients and methods:** About 3 years after disease onset, 916 rheumatoid arthritis (RA) patients of an early RA inception cohort were given a list of 32 common methods of complementary or alternative medicine (CAM) and asked whether they had used them in the previous 6 months. Differences between users and non users were explored with respect to demographic characteristics, disease severity, specialised or non specialised care, treatment and attitudes towards the health care system. **Results:** 42% of the patients had used at least one of the 32 methods; of them about half were multiple users (≥ 3 methods). Nutritional changes (30%), omission or reduction of alcohol, nicotine or coffee (27%), dietary supplements (24%) and anti-inflammatory herbal remedies (18%) were the most frequently used methods. Women had used CAM twice as often as men. There were no differences with respect to age, formal education, disease activity (DAS28), self reported disease severity and kind of treating physician. However, multiple CAM use was significantly higher in patients without DMARD therapies, in those who reported adverse effects and those who were not satisfied with the health care system. **Conclusion:** RA patients used CAM irrespectively of disease activity and of kind of care (specialised or unspecialised). CAM was most often used in addition to antirheumatic drugs. Since multiple CAM use in a small group of patients without DMARD therapy was associated with certain critical judgements regarding the health care system, this could possibly lead to insufficient treatment.

PG8-04

Heterogeneity in the use of complementary and alternative therapies (CATs) in Sweden: Exploration of committed CAT use in people with cancer

Hök J, Tishelman C, Forss A, Falkenberg T

Karolinska Institutet, Dept of Neurobiology, Care Sciences and Society, Division of Nursing, Center for Studies of Complementary Medicine, Huddinge, Sweden

Background: Research indicates that people with cancer frequently use complementary and alternative therapies (CATs). Although distinctions between different kinds of CAT usage are often not made, recent studies indicate that it can be important to further distinguish such use. Variations in CAT use have been found to be related to users' level of commitment to CAT. Further study of CAT use among committed users may contribute to a greater understanding of simultaneous use of multiple therapies. This is important knowledge for biomedically-oriented health care (BHC) and CAT providers when communicating with cancer patients about treatment choices. **Aims:** This study explores forms for committed CAT use among people with cancer. Research questions include: Which types of CATs were used? What forms of CAT use were found with regard to combinations of different therapies, providers involved and, relation to BHC treatment and cancer trajectories? Did level of commitment vary by different CAT or disease phase? **Methods:** Analysis is based on data from unstructured interviews with 40 people diagnosed with cancer reporting they had 'exceptional experiences' in relation to CAT use. Subjects volunteered for participation in response to a mass medial invitation. Inductive and quantitative data analysis was inspired by freelisting, an anthropological method used to define a domain from a particular perspective. **Results:** Preliminary analysis suggests that the US National Center for CAM (NCCAM) classifications are not sufficient to fully categorise CATs as defined by participants. For example an additional category 'Inspirational and spiritual mentors' was added, due to the essential role of these actors in the reports. All participants used multiple different CATs from several different NCCAM categories concurrently. Participants' accounts were similar in that they described lifestyle changes intertwined with CAT use as important for their health. While these trends were consistent, preliminary analysis suggests great heterogeneity in other aspects of CAT use. **Conclusion:** Preliminary analysis highlights discrepancies between professional and user definitions of CATs. Heterogeneity in CAT use among committed users with cancer, raises important methodological issues relevant for planning future CAT evaluations. Our results will be discussed with regard to implications to dialogue about CAT between patients and their providers.

PG8-05

Disclosure of complementary and alternative medicine use: The experiences of people living with cancer

Balneaves LG[1], Truant TLO[2], Kelly M[1], Brazier ASA[1], McLellan ML[3]

[1]School of Nursing, University of British Columbia, Vancouver, Canada; [2]Department of Nursing, British Columbia Cancer Agency, Canada; [3]School of Medicine, Southamptom University, UK

Background: With the growing consumer demand for information and clinical guidance related to complementary and alternative medicine (CAM), there is an increasing body of literature that focuses on strategies related to patient-provider communication about CAM. Despite recommendations for standardized CAM assessment by health professionals, patient disclosure of CAM use within the context of conventional cancer care remains sporadic. **Aims:** The objective of this study was to develop a better understanding of cancer patients' CAM disclosure experiences with conventional health professionals and CAM practitioners with the aim of developing best practice guidelines that will address possible barriers to patient-provider communication about CAM in the context of cancer care. **Methods:** A secondary data analysis was conducted using interpretative descriptive techniques on 42 interviews conducted with early and advanced stage cancer patients. **Results:** Patients described a variety of positive and negative disclosure experiences regarding CAM with conventional and complementary health professionals. Although some health professionals were perceived to be supportive and open to discussing CAM treatment options with cancer patients, other health professionals were seen as "shutting down" patients' attempts to discuss CAM through dismissive comments, lack of interest, or non-verbal behaviour. The reaction of health professionals to patients' initial disclosure of CAM use was highly influential on how and whether patients engaged their health professionals in future discussions about CAM. Only some individuals, however, reported the willingness of their health professionals to discuss CAM to influence their future CAM treatment decisions. **Conclusions:** The findings of this study will be contrasted to current guidelines related to patient-provider communication about CAM and applied to the development of recommendations for best practices related to facilitating CAM disclosure and discussion in conventional cancer care settings.

PG8-06

Knowledge, use and acceptance of complementary and alternative medicine (CAM) among elderly patients in orthopaedic rehabilitation clinics in Germany

Hapke S[1], Lüdtke R[2], Kraft K[1]

1Department of Complementary Medicine, University of Rostock, Germany; [2]Karl und Veronica Carstens Stiftung, Essen, Germany

Aims: The aim of this survey was to explore the knowledge, use and acceptance of CAM among elderly people with chronic orthopaedic diseases with special focus on geographic influences in Germany. **Methods:** In this unselective cross-sectional study a written questionnaire was handed out to 500 patients (age 50–80 years) of two orthopaedic rehabilitation clinics in East and West Germany between June and September 2005. **Results:** 84.6% of the patients returned the questionnaire. The best-known CAM treatments were acupuncture (86.3%), massage (84.6%), and hydrotherapy (73.4%). Nearly 70% of the participants treated at least one health problem with CAM in personal responsibility. Most frequently implemented types of CAMs were traditional household remedies (35.6%) and kinesiatrics (33.9%). However, only one third informed their physician about this use. In general, geographical influences were small, but for example, West Germans were more experienced with homeopathy ($p<0.01$) than East Germans. **Conclusions:** CAM is frequently used by elderly orthopaedic patients, but this is restricted to few methods. CAM options other than acupuncture, massage, hydrotherapy, kinesiatrics or household remedies were unknown to the majority of patients. Interestingly, geographically based differences, which presumably existed some 15 years ago, were not found. They may now have been levelled out.

PG8-08

Patterns and predictors of complementary and alternative therapy use in the U.S. cancer population

Fouladbakhsh J[1], Stommel M[2]

[1]College of Nursing, Wayne State University, Detroit, Michigan, USA; [2]College of Nursing, Michigan State University, USA

Significance: Complementary/alternative medicine (CAM) therapies are often used with mainstream medical treatments. Healthcare providers should understand prevalence, predictors and patterns of use and implications for patient care. **Purpose:** Determine patterns, predictors and purpose of use of CAM providers, practices and products in the U.S. cancer population in relationship to symptom management and conventional healthcare provider contact. Conceptual Framework: The CAM Healthcare Model, an extension of the Behavioral Model for Health Services Use, guided the study. Predisposing, enabling and need factors were examined for ability to predict CAM use viewed from a health service-health practice perspective (use of providers only, practices only, products only and use of combined CAM). **Methods:** A secondary analysis of the National Health Interview Survey (NHIS, 2002) using STATA 9.2 software for population estimation was conducted. The sample included individuals reporting a cancer diagnosis ($N=2262$) representing an estimated cancer population of 14.3 million. Participants reported use of 22 CAM therapies in the NHIS Alternative Health Supplement. CAM therapies were categorized as provider services, practices or products for analysis. Dependent variables included: 1) overall use of at least one CAM therapy, 2) use of specific CAM categories and 3) purpose of use (treatment/health promotion). Independent variables included: predisposing (gender, age, race, education, marital status), enabling (income, health insurance, provider-contact), and need (cancer site, symptoms, co-morbidity, health status). Analysis: Binary and Multinomial Logistic Regression were the primary statistical models used with focus on between-subject differences in CAM use. A stepwise procedure excluded potential predictor variables if p-value exceeded 0.10. **Results:** CAM use was more prevalent in the cancer population than in the non-cancer population with higher odds of use by female, middle-aged, white, and well-educated people; women were more likely to use CAM practices. Higher income, private insurance, conventional provider contact, pain and comorbidity were strong predictors of use. Data highlight the need for all healthcare providers to assess CAM use to promote quality healthcare, and to examine use within the specific categories identified in this study.

PG8-10

Psychometric properties of the ChQOL (HK version) in Hong Kong

Wong W, Lam C, Sham J, Fong LK, Fai LK, Li Z

Family Medicine Unit, Li Ka Shing Faculty of Medicine, University of Hong Kong

Background: The Chinese Quality of Life Measure (ChQOL) was developed recently in Mainland China and adapted to Hong Kong for assessing health-related quality of life (HRQOL) base on the philosophy and theory of Traditional Chinese Medicine (TCM). It has been validated and pilot tested on patient populations in Mainland China, but it has not been pilot tested in Hong Kong. **Aim:** The aim of this study was to evaluate the psychometric properties of the Chinese Quality of Life Instrument in Hong Kong, in order to determine the validity, reliability, and responsiveness of the ChQOL (HK version), in our population. **Methodology:** This is a cross-sectional, descriptive study on 569 new patients who consulted the Tung Wah Hospital Chinese Medicine General Outpatient Clinics. Each patient answered the ChQOL (HK version), the Chinese (Hong Kong) SF-36 and a structured questionnaire on socio-demography, morbidity and service utilization before the consultation with the TCM practitioner. Each subject was followed up after two weeks at the clinic or by telephone when they answered and the SF-36 again and a global rating on change of the condition. Outcome Measures: The construct validity was measured by facet-domain and domain-overall score correlations, correlations between the domain scores of the ChQOL and the SF-36. Internal reliability was measured by Cronbach's alpha. Responsiveness was measured by the change of the ChQOL scores after two weeks. **Results:** The internal consistency in all facets (Cronbach $\alpha = 0.59–0.88$) and domains (Cronbach $\alpha = 0.83–0.90$) were good. The correlation of 11 facets to 3 domains of ChQOL were high ($p<0.01$), and the 3 domains to overall of ChQOL correlation were also high which ranged from $r=0.80–0.87$, $p<0.01$. The three domains of ChQOL had moderate correlations ($r=0.33–0.65$) with the SF-36 PCS and MCS scores. Responsiveness was supported by significant improvement in all domains scores of ChQOL after 2 weeks The patients' global rating of their health status mildly correlated to the change in score of the physical form and overall health of ChQOL ($r=0.11–0.21$, $p<0.05$), which further supported its construct validity. **Conclusion:** This study supported the construct validity, reliability and responsiveness of ChQOL among patients presenting to TCM clinics in primary care. The ChQOL can be applied to clinical practice and research to complement TCM practitioner in the assessment of the effectiveness of TCM. Further research is needed to determine the clinical interpretation of the ChQOL scores.

PG8-11

Measuring the outcome of complementary and alternative medical (CAM) treatment: Symptoms versus mood versus sense of coherence

Hyland ME[1], Lewith GT[2], Wheeler P[1]

[1]Health Psychology, University of Plymouth, UK; [2]Primary Care Group, CCS Division, University of Southampton, UK

Objective: To asses if both holistic (sense of coherence and mood) and symptomatic change, during CAM treatment, follow the same patterns over time and can be measured with existing, validated scales. **Methods:** Design: An outcome study to investigate patient perceived improvement (Measure Yourself Medical Outcome Profile: MYMOP), mood (Positive and Negative Affect Scale; PANAS) and sense of coherence (SOC-3) and the relationship between these scales, over a 4 month treatment period. Patients and location: People visiting the Centre for Complementary and Integrated Medicine (CCIM, Southampton, UK) for treatment of their chronic benign illness. Outcome: Patients attending for their first appointment were recruited and completed their baseline forms (T1) at the first consultation. Three further sets of questionnaires (T2, T3 and T4) were posted with SAE to them at monthly intervals and returned to CCIM. **Results:** Forty-five patients were recruited and 40 completed the study; MYMOP ($p=0.001$), PANAS negative ($p=0.025$) and SOC-3 ($p=0.019$) all showed similar patterns of significant improvement over time; PANAS positive showed a non significant trend for improvement ($p=0.074$). **Conclusion:** CAM treatments create changes for patients beyond their main presenting symptoms and these can be sensitively measured with existing questionnaires.

PG9-01

An investigation into the practice of homeopathy and acupuncture by medical and non-medical practitioners in the UK

Majumdar A, Adams N

Faculty of Health and Applied Social Sciences, Liverpool John Moores University, UK

Background: Acupuncture and homeopathy are two of the most widely practiced CAM therapies in Europe. Much debate surrounds these therapies both in terms of their effectiveness for different conditions and on the way they are practiced. The degree of integration of CAM therapies into the conventional medical system varies throughout Europe and integration of CAM into the NHS of the UK is a heavily debated topic. **Aim:** In order to evaluate homeopathy and acupuncture practice in the UK and to add to the debate on who should practice CAM, in what setting and using which methods, this study investigated the practices and views of medical and non-medical practitioners. **Methods:** Acupuncturists and homeopaths affiliated to the British Acupuncture Council, British Medical Acupuncture Council, Acupuncture Association of Chartered Physiotherapists, Faculty of Homeopaths and Society of Homeopaths were surveyed. Practitioners based in four regions of the UK were randomly selected from the registers of the affiliations mentioned, n=1200 and surveyed by post. Responses were analysed using SPSS. In addition qualitative data was obtained from the survey using open questions and also from some follow-up interviews. **Results:** Analysis of the study is on-going. Preliminary results highlighted significant differences between medical and non-medical practitioners including practice of other CAM, opinions on theories of the underlying mechanisms by which treatments worked and views of other medicine systems. In particular, conventional medicine was viewed more favorably by medical homeopaths ($p= 0.0001$) and Traditional Chinese Medicine was considered more favorably by non-medical acupuncturists ($p=0.0001$). Practitioners reported presentation of the same conditions, though the degree to which practitioners felt their treatments were effective for these conditions varied, with non-medical practitioners more strongly in agreement that their treatments were effective for skin diseases (homeopaths $p =0.023$), asthma (homeopaths $p=0.0006$, acupuncturists $p=0.003$) and digestive disorders (acupuncturists $p= 0.001$) than medical acupuncturists and homeopaths. **Conclusion:** The results of this study will be useful in future design methodology of studies on acupuncture and homeopathy and are also of interest in the debate of integration of CAM therapies.

PG9-02

What do physicians interested in complementary therapies think about clinical research – a survey

Icsezer S, Linde K

Center for Complementary Medicine Research, Technical University Munich, Germany

Background: In Germany a great number of physicians undergo postgraduate training in complementary therapies. We investigated to what extent participants of courses on complementary therapies consider clinical research relevant. **Methods:** Two-hundred-fifty (63% female, mean age 39.9 (SD 7.0) years) physicians participating in official postgraduate teaching programs for homeopathy (n = 96), acupuncture (n = 79) and naturopathy (n = 75) were asked to fill in a 4-page questionnaire with questions on their general attitudes toward research, the relevance of research for practice, and how they keep up to date. **Results:** Participants of homeopathy courses were more often female (77% versus 54% in the acupuncture and 53% in the naturopathy courses; $p<0.01$), had a higher age on average (42.5 years vs. 38.2 and 38.2 years; $p<0.01$), worked less often in a hospital (21% vs. 45% vs. 35%; $p < 0.01$), and already used complementary therapies more often (61% vs. 23% vs. 40%; $p<0.01$). Clinical research was considered of high/very high relevance by 34%/18% of participants in the homeopathy, 55%/13% in the acupuncture and 53%/14% in the naturopathy courses ($p=0.08$). 30% vs. 28% vs. 45% reported that they base the majority of clinical decisions on evidence from clinical research ($p=0.07$). 56% of homeopathy, 48%

of acupuncture and 44% of naturopathy (p=0.68) course participants agree to the statement that trials rarely are directly applicable to clinical practice. More than ninety percent in all three groups agreed to the statement that they would to try to keep up to date with current research findings if they would have a strategy that would cost only 15 minutes per week. **Conclusion:** Physicians undergoing postgraduate training in homeopathy in Germany seem to be more sceptical about the relevance of clinical research for their practice than physicians participating in acupuncture or naturopathy courses.

PG9-03

Representation of complementary and alternative medicine for cancer in the Canadian print media

Weeks L[1], Verhoef M[1], Scott C[1, 2]

[1]Department of Community Health Sciences, University of Calgary, Canada; [2]Calgary Health Region, Canada

Aims: Cancer patients repeatedly identify mass media as primary information sources influencing their decisions regarding complementary and alternative medicine (CAM) use. The necessarily incomplete nature of media reports raises concerns regarding the accuracy, balance and quality of the information upon which many patients make decisions. This study aims to determine: 1) what is reported in the Canadian print media regarding CAM treatment for cancer; 2) how that information is represented; and 3) trends in reporting frequency and reporting characteristics. **Methods:** A content analysis is being conducted on 1,150 articles published between Jan/1990 and Dec/2005 in popular Canadian newspapers and magazines. A coding template includes: types of CAM; cancer type; topics covered (e.g., risks, benefits); sources of evidence used in text; recommendations made regarding use, access and discussions with healthcare providers; and article prominence (e.g., number of words). The analysis will be primarily descriptive (e.g., frequencies, mean). Group comparisons will identify differences by media type (e.g., chi-squared statistics). Trends in reporting frequency and characteristics will be sought and compared with corresponding trends in CAM use as reported in the literature during this period. **Results:** This research is in progress. Preliminary results suggest annual trends in reporting frequency correspond to trends in CAM use. Trends in annual reporting frequency do not differ proportionally by therapy type. The most frequently referred to therapies are: natural health products, CAM therapies in general, nutrition (including special diets), meditation, spirituality and yoga. Again, reporting frequency corresponds to documented use. Further results to address complete study aims will be available for May/2007. **Conclusions:** Preliminary results confirm the persuasive role of the media in CAM decision making, but raise the question of exactly how CAM use relates to CAM coverage. This study is part of a larger study that will further explore and improve this relationship by helping patients to critically appraise media information and journalists to represent more accurate, balanced and complete information.

PG9-04

A step towards introducing complementary and alternative medicine in problem based learning curriculum

Sachdeva U

Department of Physiology, College of Medicine and Medical Sciences, Arabian Gulf University, Bahrain

Background: The current increase in use, research and documentation of Complementary and Alternative Medicine (CAM) has generated increased attention of medical educators. Many medical schools around the world are now including CAM courses in their primary core curriculum. Yet in Gulf region such initiative has not taken place. **Objective:** To solicit the opinion of medical students about their attitude and inclusion of elements of CAM in medical curriculum, and compare this after exposure to familiarization course in a PBL curriculum. **Methods:** Study design and subjects: In phase I of the study a survey was conducted on medical students (n=200) of various medical schools of Gulf region, by giving them a pre-tested questionnaire to assess their knowledge, attitude and acceptance for inclusion of CAM in medical curriculum. Following this a task force of 10 faculty members of PBL School framed a short educational plan for clerkship students (Year 5-6), in the form of case-based series of 3 workshops. At the end of course the questionnaire was re-administered. The comparison pre and post scores given by Likert Scale were statistically analyzed. **Results:** The students were only aware of 3 out of 10 CAM modalities listed in the questionnaire. After the workshop there was no significant change in their awareness grading. However a significant ($p<.05$) increase was reported in the area of acceptance to seek more information. There was modest increase ($p<.05$) in mean score of willingness and domain for inclusion of CAM in curriculum was recorded. There was shift in opinion for educational method for learning of CAM from elective to formal courses. **Conclusion:** The results suggest that senior medical students had a desire to include CAM in PBL curriculum as formal courses. The short familiarization courses are not sufficient to increase their knowledge of CAM but only serve as vehicle for increasing their interest for learning.

PG9-05

Holistic thinking in basic sciences and medicine – needs assessment and experimental pilot-course for medical students at the University of Berne

Heusser P, Wolf U

Institute of Complementary Medicine, University of Berne, Switzerland

Background: Integration of complementary and alternative medicine (CAM) into academic medicine necessitates an evidence based approach to demonstrate its effectiveness, but also a scientifically justifiable account of its basic tenets such as holistic thinking (HT). Since patients often experience and welcome HT as an attribute of CAM which is lacking in conventional medicine it should be integrated into medical education. **Aims:** 1) To assess the need for holistic thinking among medical students at the University of Berne; 2) to develop a credit rewarded elective on holistic thinking, and 3) to pilot and evaluate the course. **Methods:** 1) A survey was carried out assess needs for education in holistic thinking among all 1st and 2nd year medical students of 2004/05. 2) A 20 hour elective course was developed on the principles of Goethe's holistic Empiric Rationalism and applied to basic topics of epistemology, physics, chemistry, molecular biology, morphology, sensory physiology, mind-body issues and ethics. Integration with core curricular content was sought. A selection of eight hours was taught as a pilot course with a group of 6 students. 3) At the end, a questionnaire was filled out by students to evaluate course elements, instruction, subjectively perceived cognitive and emotional learner objectives. **Results:** 1) The return rate for the survey was 50% (193/394), of whom 99% indicated that physicians should be able to think holistically, 90% that holistic thinking should be taught in medical education, and 54% that they might inscribe in such a course. 2) Among the 6 students of the pilot course, global course acceptance was high (mean global rate of 5.2, range 5-6, on a 6-point scale), and so was the acceptance of course elements, instruction, affective satisfaction with the course, judgment of cognitive course aspects and of the scientific justification of the holistic concepts discussed. However, students felt in part overcharged with the intellectual competency addressed, the quantity of content and the pace of its delivery. **Conclusions:** 1) The survey showed a need for holistic thinking in medical education. 2) The new elective course seems to provide a well accepted and scientifically reasonable approach to HT in basic sciences and medicine, but improvements are necessary. The results of this pilot study encourage us to implement the course.

PG9-06

Content validity of the integrative medicine attitude questionnaire: Perspectives of Hong Kong Chinese expert panel

Chung V, Wong E, Griffiths S

School of Public Health, Chinese University of Hong Kong

Objective: The increasing popularity of Complementary and Alternative Medicine (CAM) amongst patients and the public and moves to integrate different practice modalities amongst physicians requires a greater understanding. Whilst the Integrative Medicine Attitude Questionnaire (IMAQ) is a validated instrument developed in the US for measuring allopathic physicians' attitude towards CAM, little is known about attitudes amongst western trained doctors in other societies particularly in the Far East. In Hong Kong, cultural and historical forces have created a unique environment for integration. Thus consideration of such forces suggests that direct use of the original IMAQ for assessing attitudes of allopathic physicians' views on traditional Chinese medicine (TCM) in Hong Kong would be inappropriate. This hypothesis was tested using content validity judgement and local experts' opinions, to assess the three domains of IMAQ: "holism", "introspection and doctor-patient relationship", and "effectiveness of integrative treatment". **Methods:** Standard content validity establishment methodologies were followed. An eight member panel (four with TCM & four with allopathic medicine backgrounds) was convened to assess the content validity of a modified HK TCM specific IMAQ. Experts were provided with explicit instructions on how to evaluate the content validity of individual items, and the instrument as a whole, both quantitatively and qualitatively. **Results:** Out of 28 items, 12 items of the modified IMAQ were content validity adequate (Content validity Index (CVI) > 0.70 and kappa > 0.4). Seven items were considered content invalid and removed. The overall CVI and kappa of the instrument was 0.71 and 0.09 respectively, indicating the need to modify 9 marginally valid items which remained in the questionnaire. Qualitative expert comments were used for the revision. **Conclusion:** The process of validation showed that it would be inappropriate for the US derived IMAQ to be used without modification in Hong Kong. Most of the content valid items were in the "effectiveness of integrative treatment" domain, which reflected the influence of the evidence based TCM movement on the experts' judgement. Further development and validation of the instrument by factor analysis is warranted and studies are planned.

PG9-07

Evaluation of bilingual self-learning modules on website for complementary/alternative medicine practitioners and health professionals

Blanchet C, Cauchon M, Labrecque M, Marc I, Ernst E, Dodin S

Lucie et André Chagnon Chair's for the teaching of an integrated approach in prevention, Faculty of medicine, Laval University, Quebec, Canada

Objective: The aim of this project was to evaluate three bilingual self-learning website modules intended for CAM practitioners and health professionals. The objective of this website was to offer methodological tools in order to develop good ability of researching valid information and encourage the development of a systematic approach of CAM literature. **Materials and method:** All modules were based on clinical situations that refer to the use of CAM. French and English CAM practitioners or health professionals evaluate the three modules. They got through them in a specific order; module 1) How to find information that is pertinent and valid, module 2) Evaluation of an article on a complementary or alternative therapy to prevention or treatment, and module 3) Exploring the question from all angles: review article, systematic reviews and meta-analyses. After each module, a questionnaire was completed evaluate the pedagogical aspects, virtual presentation and navigation on the web. Also, few questions were added in order to evaluate knowledge modifications after the lecture of each module. **Results:** The French evaluators found that the site offered a potential of abundant scientific research and allowed them to obtain information from conventional medicine. Overall, the content of each module seemed good enough to bring new knowledge or to push them further. The majority of them would recommend these self-learning modules to colleagues. In regards of the English evaluators, the results are still being compiled and will be presented in the poster. **Conclusion:** The three French self-learning modules led CAM practitioners or health professionals to discover and use in a progressive, educative and practical way various resources available on the internet and provide adequate information about CAM. Acknowledgement: Funded by Health Canada.

PG10-01

The Rosen method body work - an exploratory study of an uncharted complementary therapy

Hoffrén-Larsson R[1], Falkenberg T[2]

[1]Dept. of Neurobiology, Care Sciences and Society, Division of Nursing; [2]Center for Studies of Complementary Medicine (CSC), Karolinska Institutet, Stockholm, Sweden

Aim: This study examines the Rosen Method body work, a complementary therapy practise that has gained in interest during the last decade. Despite many informal reports on successful treatments there are no scientific studies on the method. Therefore, the aim of this study is to obtain initial knowledge of the Rosen method: 1) Why do clients consult the Rosen Method? 2) What is the clients' self reported "quality of health"? and 3) What experiences do the clients report? **Methods:** In this exploratory study 65 Swedish clients under treatment (average 27 sessions) answered two questionnaires. The first survey contained 20 items focusing on the reasons for consulting the Rosen Method and earlier experiences from conventional medicine. These data were analysed descriptively. The second questionnaire measured "quality of health" using Quola SF-36. The data were compared with answers from a representative sample (sex and age matched) of the Swedish population, and analysed with Mann-Whitney U-test. **Results:** The self reported reasons for consulting the method were complex, involving both severe physical and psychological health problems (e.g. bodily pain, muscular tensions, stress and other psychological causes). Eighty-six percent reported these problems to be markedly bothersome in their daily life, and forty-five percent had consulted conventional medicine for help. Clients´ "quality of health" was significantly lower than the average population in four of the eight SF-36 scales. Seventy-three percent reported that the Rosen Method helped them in a high or very high degree which was in contrast to their experience from conventional care. Almost every client reported considerable health effects of the treatment. The effects were of primary physical (e.g. less pain and muscle tensions) or psychological character (e.g. feeling less moody). In addition, health promoting effects were reported due to the clients own behavioral changes. **Conclusions:** Clients report that they consult the Rosen Method for severe health problems and experience multi-dimensional positive effects of the treatments. Further research is needed to investigate what in the treatment situation leads to the positive health effects reported.

PG10-02

The effect of acoustic stimuli on heart-rate variability

Kratky KW, Diepold D, Schaefer A

Working Group "Physics of Physiological Processes", University of Vienna, Austria

Introduction: Acoustic stimuli can cause changes in physiological variables, which are reflected in heart-rate variability (HRV). Due to the analysis of HRV, statements concerning the regulatory state of the autonomic nervous system and the circulatory system are possible. We investigated the effect of acoustic stimuli on HRV variables. **Experiments and methods:** This work was concerned with the effect of three different acoustic stimuli ("pink noise", "water", "frogs"), coming from a CD with a sound pressure level of 70 dB(A). Twelve healthy volunteers took part in the experiments (6 women and men each). The age of the test persons ranged between 22 and 27 years. The test persons listened to the acoustic stimuli for 15 minutes. The exposition to the stimuli was preceded and followed by 15 minutes of silence. During the periods of acoustic irradiation and silence, HRV was measured two times each for a length of 300 heartbeats. These measurements started 2 and 9.5 minutes after the beginning of the respective periods. The aim of this work was to investigate if significant differences of the HRV variables occur between periods of acoustic irradiation and silence. Evaluation included time- and frequency-domain variables, nonlinear measures and pulse-respiration variables. **Results:** "Frogs" caused the most pronounced differences with respect to the HRV variables. Significant results were observed for specific time- and frequency-domain variables and nonlinear measures, as well as for breathing rate and pulse-respiration quotient. The stimulus "water" showed significant differences for specific frequency-domain and for nonlinear measures. "Pink noise" caused significant results only for one variable that is closely connected with the heart rate itself. **Conclusions:** The results show that acoustic stimuli can influence HRV within minutes and that the effects of individual stimuli can be distinguished by HRV analysis. It is interesting to note that the artificial "pink noise" has fewer effects than the more natural "frogs" and "water". This may be compared with an analogous result of an anterior study where expositions to full-spectrum and commercial neutral white fluorescent light were compared. The effects on HRV variables were more pronounced for the more natural full-spectrum light.

PG10-03

Efficacy of neural therapy in referred patients with chronic pain

Fischer L, Pfister M

Institute of Complementary Medicine, University of Berne, Switzerland

Aims: The effectiveness of the neural therapeutic treatment was investigated in patients with chronic pain after a long-term observation regarding the outcomes pain and medication use. Due to an increase in referrals of chronic pain patients (N=72) to neural therapy, we decided to perform a clinical study including all referred patients over three years. Neural therapy according to Huneke is a treatment, which uses injections with local anaesthetics for diagnosis and therapy. Neural therapy is based on neurophysiological stimulation and inhibition mechanisms which can be applied therapeutically. **Methods:** All referred pain patients between 2001 and 2004 were included in the study. Patients suffered from severe chronic pain (most frequently backache), which showed a therapy resistance for conventional (medication, physical therapy, operations etc.) and complementary (e.g. acupuncture, homeopathy) therapies. They had chronic pain for on average 6.2 (standard deviation: 7.5) years before the referral. **Results:** Patients needed on average 8 (standard deviation: 7.7) neural therapeutic treatments. The most significant improvement occurred after 3.7 (standard deviation: 4.0) consultations. One fifth of the patients remained therapy resistant, one third showed a significant improvement, one quarter was free of pain after several months. 60% of patients could reduce their medication (observation time of several months). **Conclusions:** Neural therapy shows good long-term results in the majority of chronic pain patients with therapy resistance to conventional treatments. On the basis of these results we plan a prospective clinical study with chronic pain patients.

PG10-04

Static magnetic field therapy: A critical assessment of reported dosing regimens

Colbert A, Wahbeh H, Harling N, Connelly E, Forsten C, Schiffke H, Gregory W, King V, Markov M, Elmer P

The Helfgott Research Institute at the National College of Natural Medicine, Portland, USA

Aims: Despite widespread consumer use of permanent magnets and numerous clinical trials of static magnetic field (SMF) therapy, there are few well designed Phase I/II studies that have optimized the physical and biophysical parameters of SMF dosimetry. A lack of understanding or reporting the physical parameters of the permanent magnet that generates the therapeutic SMF may lead to inappropriate conclusions regarding SMF effectiveness. The purpose of this review is to appraise dosing regimens reported in published SMF studies and to offer preliminary guidelines for designing a scientifically based SMF clinical trial. **Methods:** Human clinical studies (excluding animal studies, abstracts, posters, and editorials) using therapeutic SMFs were sought in electronic databases and reference lists. Also excluded were studies reporting on combination therapies, electromagnetic fields, transcranial magnetic stimulation, and magnets on acupuncture points. Data on 11 essential dosing parameters were extracted including: name of target tissue; magnet dimensions, materials, field strength, pole configuration; site, frequency, duration and method of application, distance of magnet surface from target; and rationale for use of a specific magnet. A quality assessment (QA) score was calculated for reporting these 11 essential dosing parameters. Two points were given if a parameter was fully described, one point if partially described and 0 points if not described. **Results:** Fifty-five SMF studies were identified. Thirteen were conducted in healthy volunteers and 42 in patient populations. No study received a perfect QA score of 22. Only eighteen studies (32%) scored 17–22; 49% scored 11–16: 16% scored 6–10 and one scored 0–5. The dosing parameter most often reported was frequency of magnet application (93%). Least often reported was distance of the magnet surface from the target tissue (11%). 78% of studies failed to provide enough information about dosing parameters to determine whether the SMF was sufficient to reach the target tissue. **Conclusions:** Findings from this project highlight the need to precede full scale randomized controlled trials with Phase II studies in which SMF dosing parameters are optimized. Guidelines are outlined for choosing a magnet with the essential physical and biophysical characteristics necessary to generate a SMF that is adequate to reach the target tissue.

PG10-05

Long-term efficacy of Okada purifying therapy (bio-energy healing) on menopausal women

Suzuki K[1,2], Hatayama M[2], Ishida A[2], Torii H[2], Uchida S[1], Tanaka C[2], Kaizuka S[2]

[1]MOA Health Science Foundation; [2]Tokyo Ryo-in MOA Takanawa Clinic, Japan

Aims: Complementary and alternative therapies for menopausal women are gaining popularity. Okada purifying therapy (OPT) is bio-energy healing modality used for health promotion; however, its clinical efficacy is still unknown. The purpose of this pilot study was to determine whether symptoms around menopause improve with frequent OPT practice. **Methods:** In 127 menopausal women, 25 received daily OPT for 3 months, 35 received regular practice (more than biweekly), and 67 underwent less frequent OPT from the certified practitioners. The change of symptoms evaluated with Kupperman's index was compared among the groups. In those receiving daily practice, we also examined the heart rate variability, female hormones and psychological states. **Results:** Daily OPT practice improved their symptoms significantly (from 34±14 to 14±13, $p<0.001$) even in the face of continued hormonal imbalance. Regular practice was less effective than daily OPT (from 35±11 to 26±13, $p=0.003$), and less frequent OPT did not improve the symptoms. Moreover, frequent OPT (more than every other day) stabilized the symptoms for 3 years (23±14 vs 31±14, $p=0.001$). Analyses of heart rate variability suggested that OPT activated the parasympathetic nerve (from 0.94±0.34 to 1.25±0.43 msec/Hz1/2, $p=0.001$), except in one patient with over-stimulated activity, and suppressed the sympathetic nerve (from 10.87±4.75 to 8.11±4.16, $p=0.023$). **Conclusions:** Frequent Okada purifying therapy improved menopausal symptoms to a greater extent, probably due to influencing the autonomic nerve activity.

PG10-06

The training and support programme for parents of children with cerebral palsy

Cheshire A, Barlow J, Powell L

Coventry University, UK

Aims: The Training and Support Programme (TSP) was designed to improve the psychosocial well-being of parents of children with disabilities by teaching parents how to massage their child. Previous research has demonstrated that following the TSP parents of children with disabilities showed significant improvements in parental self-efficacy for managing their child's psychosocial well-being, parental self-efficacy for giving their child massage and significant reductions in parental levels of anxiety. The purpose of this study was to evaluate the efficacy of the TSP with a more homogeneous group, parents of children with cerebral palsy (CP). **Methods:** The study utilized a pre-post test design. Forty-three participants were recruited via voluntary organisations, special schools and health professionals. Questionnaires comprising standard measures of quality of life and parental perceptions' of child's functioning were mailed to participants at two points in time, baseline (immediately pre-Programme) and at 4-month follow-up. **Results:** The majority of parents were mothers (88.4%), were married or living with a partner (88.4%), White European (81.4%) and had educational qualifications (95.3%). Parents had a mean age of 40 (SD=7) years. Comparisons between study variables at baseline and 4-month follow-up revealed a significant reduction in parental anxious mood (p=0.018) and perceived stress (p=0.030), and a significant increase in satisfaction with life (p=0.009). There were trends towards improvement on depressed mood (p=0.082) and parents' self-efficacy for managing children's psychosocial well-being (p=0.068). There were significant improvements in parental perceptions' of children's sleeping (p=0.005), mobility (p=0.0005) and verbal communication (p=0.034). There was a trend towards improvement in children's eating (p=0.081). There were no significant changes on generalised self-efficacy, parental health status, self-efficacy for massage and children's non-verbal communication. **Conclusion:** For parents of children with CP, the TSP appears to have a positive effect on parental psychosocial well-being and child functioning.

PG10-07

Development of a new massage therapy diagnostic assessment

Baskwill A, Finch P, Dryden T
Centennial College, Toronto, Canada

Background: It is known that there are internationally educated health care professionals residing in Canada who face barriers to entering practice. Reducing these barriers has become a government priority. In this context, the College of Massage Therapists of Ontario (CMTO) initiated a project to develop an assessment process and bridging program for internationally educated massage therapists (IEMTs). As a result, the Massage Therapy Diagnostic Assessment was created and first administered in November 2006. **Objective:** The objective of this diagnostic assessment is to evaluate the knowledge and skills of IEMTs who wish to practice in Ontario. Based on the results of this process recommendations are made to each candidate regarding which of the various options (immediate access to CMTO certification examination, bridging program, diploma program), s/he would be advised to pursue. **Description of the Diagnostic Assessment:** The Massage Therapy Diagnostic Assessment consisted of three components: a multiple-choice health science exam, an objectively structured clinical examination (OSCE), and a comprehensive clinical evaluation. The combination of these components allows for sufficient demonstration of knowledge and skills associated with the practice competencies related to massage therapy in Ontario. The OSCE was evaluated using competency checklists. The comprehensive clinical evaluation was evaluated using Finch's Intervention Zones. **Results:** The information that was gathered about each candidate as a result of the assessment process was impressive. Upon completion of the diagnostic assessment, a profile was created for each candidate outlining his/her areas of strength and areas needing further education. Recommendations were then made to the candidates with regard to the amount of further education needed in order to be prepared for the entry-to-practice examinations offered by the College of Massage Therapists of Ontario. **Recommendations:** It is recommended that this process be considered for other health care professions. It would be especially beneficial for those professions in which credentialing of candidates is not straightforward or where a specific proficiency in knowledge or skills is needed to enter a program/ course.

PG10-08

Traditional medicine in the Creole population of Belize, Central America

Ives R
The College of Osteopaths, UK

Aims: An exploratory study to record the existence and use of traditional manual healing methods within the Creole population of Belize. The tiny English-speaking country of Belize is situated in Central America, surrounded by Latin speaking countries. Its highly diverse biology and geography has made it an emerging centre for eco-tourism. Its human population is culturally diverse with at least six different ethnic populations, including the Creoles and indigenous Mayans. Creole inhabitants of the remote villages of the southern part of the country rely heavily on traditional methods of healing. **Methods:** Data were collected through a wide-ranging document search, interviews, and ethnographic observation. Subjects were healers and members of the Creole population recruited through a knowledgeable local Creole contact. **Results:** Document sources contained few clues to the healing traditions in Belize. Tourist information led to discovery of a book written by a western naturopath on the healing traditions of the Mayan Indian community, but no information was found on the Creole traditions. Interviews were conducted in their therapeutic settings with two manual healers, a bush doctor, a midwife, and with members of the user population. Considerable emphasis on fertility, pregnancy and childbirth was found both in practitioners and the population. Manipulative and visceral manual methods were widely used, and a "hands-on" practice called "nine-ting" was mentioned by several subjects. **Discussion:** This was the first study in this area. The villages studied are remote and poor and the research was aided by the availability of a local contact and the readiness of the people to share information verbally. Healing in Belize appeared to be culture-specific and used widely in the village population for regulating fertility. People would travel many miles to visit one of the few healers of their own culture. The indigenous healing tradition is unwritten and handed down by word of mouth. **Conclusions:** Further research is needed to gather further information on the unique "nineting" and other manual techniques, and to understand how healers are chosen and how they practice.

Forschende
Komplementärmedizin
Wissenschaft • Praxis • Perspektiven

Author Index

Forsch Komplementärmed 2007;14(suppl 1):54–55

KARGER

Fax +49 761 4 52 07 14
E-mail Information@Karger.de
www.karger.com

Accessible online at:
www.karger.com/fok

Forschende Komplementärmedizin
Wissenschaft • Praxis • Perspektiven

Guidelines for Authors

Forsch Komplementärmed 2007;14

Submission
'Research in Complementary Medicine' is a peer-reviewed journal that publishes articles written in German or English on basic research, clinical studies, methodology or scientific theory in complementary medicine.
Manuscripts can be submitted online at *www.karger.com/fok*.
Should you have any problems with electronic submission, or feel the need to submit the paper in a non-electronic form, please send your manuscript to:

S. Karger Verlag für Medizin und Naturwissenschaften GmbH
Attn.: Dipl.-Psych. Franziska Lang
P.O. Box
79095 Freiburg (Germany)
Tel. +49 761 45 20 726
Fax +49 761 45 20 714
E-mail f.lang@karger.de

Types of Papers and Allotted Number of Pages
Manuscripts should be written double-spaced, 12-point size, with 3-cm margins. Please use only one format (normal) for the document.
Contributions are classified as: Original Article, Review Article, Case Report, Essay, Methodology, Documentation, Editorial, Journal Club, Congress Report, Book Review, Letter to the Editors. Articles should not exceed 8 printed pages (case reports: 4). Short communications of scientific results should not exceed 3 printed pages. (As a rule of thumb, 3 manuscript pages, including cover sheet, tables, figures are equal to 1 printed page.) Each additional complete or partial page to print will be charged to the author.

Reports on Randomized Controlled Trials (RCTs) should be prepared according to the CONSORT statement [Begg C, Cho M, Eastwood S, Horton S, Moher D, Olki I, Pitkin R, Rennie D, Schulz F, Simel D, Stroup D: Improving the quality of reporting of randomized trials: The CONSORT statement. JAMA 1996;276:637–639]. The report must state explicitly how the comparison groups were assembled, allowing the reader to access the method of randomization. Please specify in the title and summary that the manuscript is a report on an RCT. When an RCT is submitted, the authors should refer to the 'Checklist for Authors Submitting Randomized Controlled Trials' available at *http://www.consort-statement.org*. Both should be submitted with the manuscript, as they will be included in the review process.
Reports on homeopathic treatments should be prepared according to the RedHot-Supplement to CONSORT [Dean ME, Coulter MK, Fisher P, Jobst K, Walach H: Reporting data on homeopathic treatments (RedHot): A supplement to CONSORT. Forsch Komplementärmed 2006;13:368–371].

Conditions
Acceptance of a manuscript is based on the evaluation by several reviewers (peer review).
Manuscripts are received with the explicit understanding that they are not under simultaneous consideration by any other publication. Submission of an article for publication implies the transfer of the copyright from the author to the publisher upon acceptance.
Once the manuscript is accepted for publication, all usage rights will be retained by the publisher. The assignment of usage rights applies to all print media as well as electronic offline and online media, including the Internet and data bases/data carriers of any kind. Accepted papers, in whole or in part, may not be translated into other languages, or reproduced by any mechanical or electronic means (including photocopying, recording and microcopying), or stored in a retrieval system without the written consent of the publisher.
It is the authors' responsibility to obtain permission to produce illustrations, tables, etc. from other publications.
All forms of support, including that from drug companies, and any potential source of conflict of interest should be acknowledged in the cover letter to the editor. Should the manuscript be accepted, the editor will discuss the extent of disclosure appropriate for publication with the authors. The publisher reserves the right to edit the manuscript and decide on the layout.

Ethical and Legal Prerequisites
Manuscripts involving examinations of probands and patents must include a statement that the trial protocol has been approved by an ethical committee and thus meets the standards of the Declaration of Helsinki in its revised version of 1975 and its amendments of 1983, 1989, and 1996 [JAMA 1997;277:925–926]. Accordingly, the proband's informed consent has to be mentioned in the manuscript. Information suitable to reveal the proband's identity is to be avoided.
Experiments involving animals demand consent as well and must meet the requirements of German laws for the protection of animals in their current version. A reference to this approval must be included in the manuscript. Articles from countries other than Germany must include a comparable note.

Arrangement
Authors' affiliations and address of correspondence: Each author's full name, followed by their affiliation (hospital, institute etc. where the work was conducted) and the exact postal address of the corresponding author complete with postal code must be given in a separate document to allow a blind review process. Please also supply phone and fax numbers, as well as e-mail address.

Title page: The first page of each paper should indicate the title (in German **and** English) and a short title for use as running head.

Key Words: For indexing purposes, a list of 3-5 key words in English and German is essential. Whenever possible, use key words such as found in the Medical Subject Headings List (MeSH) of Index Medicus.

Summary: Summaries must be submitted in German and English. They must not exceed 250 words each. Summaries of Original Articles should be structured as follows: Background (or Introduction), Patients and Methods (or Material and Methods), Results, Conclusion.

Footnotes: Footnotes should be used only for tables.

Registered Trade Names: When first mentioned, registered trade names must be marked with the superscript registration symbol ® or ™. It is the sole responsibility of the author to ensure that this rule is followed properly.

Tables and Illustrations: Tables and illustrations should be prepared on separate sheets. *Tables* require a heading and figures a legend, also prepared on a separate sheet. The number of figures and tables should be limited and aim to illustrate the text. Figures are listed in the text as (fig. 1), tables as (table 1). Data already mentioned in the text need not be repeated in a table. Accordingly, numbers used in tables need not be repeated in the text.
For the reproduction of *illustrations*, only good drawings and original photographs can be accepted. On the back of each illustration, indicate its number, the author's name, and 'top' with a soft pencil. Electronically submitted b/w half-tone and color illustrations must have a final resolution of 300 dpi after scaling, line drawings one of 800–1200 dpi.
Color illustrations are reproduced at the author's expense. Each one is charged to the author at EUR 260.– + VAT as contribution to the additional reproduction and color printing costs.

References
The list of **references** should include only the publications cited in the text. References must be numbered sequentially in the order cited in the text. In the text identify references by Arabic numerals [in square brackets]. In each reference at least the first 3 authors should be named. It is recommended to quote only articles already published or accepted for publication. Please avoid 'in preparation' or 'personal communication'. Authors are responsible for the accuracy and completeness of their references and for correct citation. Journal titles should be abbreviated according to the Index Medicus system (www.nlm.nih.gov). If a reference manager is used, the style «Pharmacology» or «Nephron» should be chosen.
Examples for references:

Papers published in periodicals:
1 Lelie PN, Cuypers HTM, van Drimmelen AAJ, Quint WGV: Quality assessment of hepatitis C virus nucleic acid amplification methods. An international proficiency study. Infusionsther Transfusionsmed 1998;25:102–110.

Papers published only with DOI numbers:
2 Theoharides TC, Boucher W, Spear K: Serum interleukin-6 reflects disease severity and osteoporosis in mastocytosis patients. Int Arch Allergy Immunol DOI: 10.1159/000063858.

Papers published in electronic format:
3 Black CA: Delayed type hypersensitivity: Current theories with a historic perspective. Dermatol Online J 1999;5:7. http://dermatology.dclib.org/DOJvol5num1.

Edited books:
4 Hardy WD Jr, Essex M: FeLV-induced feline acquired immune deficiency syndrome: A model for human AIDS; in Klein E (ed): Acquired Immunodeficiency Syndrome. Prog Allergy. Basel, Karger, 1986, vol 37, pp 353–376.

Monographs:
5 Schaefer UW, Beelen DW: Bone Marrow Transplantation, ed 2, revised. Basel, Karger, 1996.

Page Charges
There are no page charges for papers that do not exceed the allotted size (cf. types of papers). Each additional complete or partial page is charged to the author at 365.– EUR + VAT.

Galley Proofs
Unless indicated otherwise, galley proofs are sent to the corresponding author and should be returned with the least possible delay. Alterations made in galley proofs, other than the correction of printer's errors, are charged to the author. No page proofs are supplied.

Reprints
Order forms and a price list are sent with the galley proofs. Orders submitted after the issue is printed are subject to considerably higher prices.

KARGER
Fax +49 761 4 52 07 14
E-mail Information@Karger.de
www.karger.com

Guidelines for Authors available at:
www.karger.com/fok_gl.htm

Internationale Zeitschrift für Grundlagenforschung, klinische Prüfungen, Methodologie, Praxis und Wissenschaftstheorie

Forschende Komplementärmedizin

Wissenschaft • Praxis • Perspektiven

Research in Complementary Medicine

Research • Practice • Perspectives

Offizielles Organ der Schweizerischen Medizinischen Gesellschaft für Phytotherapie

Offizielles Organ der European Society for Complementary and Natural Medicine

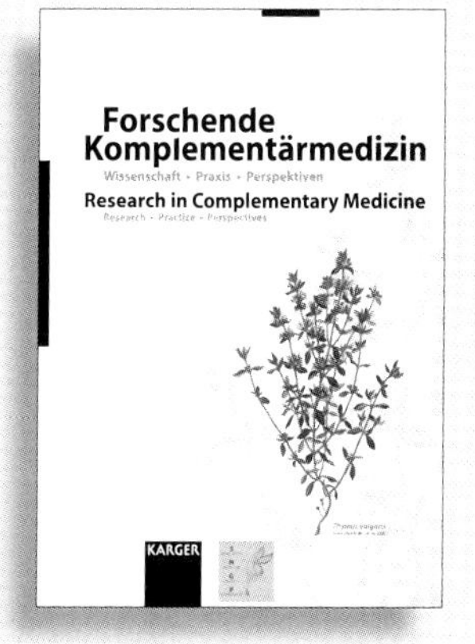

Hauptschriftleitung

H. Walach, Northampton

Fachschriftleitung

R. Lüdtke, Essen
P.F. Matthiessen, Herdecke
D. Melchart, München
K.M. Meyer-Abich, Hamburg
A. Michalsen, Essen
B. Reiter, Wien
K.L. Resch, Bad Elster
R. Saller, Zürich
C. Witt, Berlin

Forschende Komplementärmedizin ist eine internationale Zeitschrift, die auf wissenschaftlicher Ebene Brücken zwischen Schul- und Komplementärmedizin baut und somit die Integration dieser beiden Bereiche fördert. Entsprechend arbeiten im wissenschaftlichen Beirat Schul- und Alternativmediziner verschiedener Disziplinen zusammen. Sie entscheiden aufgrund eines differenzierten Review-Verfahrens über die Annahme der wissenschaftlichen Beiträge, um eine hohe Qualität der Publikationen zu gewährleisten. Daneben werden regelmässig wichtige neue Publikationen aus internationalen Fachzeitschriften vorgestellt und von Experten kommentiert.

Eine Auswahl repräsentativer Beiträge

Acupuncture in the Treatment of Painful Dysfunction of the Temporomandibular Joint – a Review of the Literature: **Fink, M.** (Hannover); **Rosted, P.** (Sheffield); **Bernateck, M.; Stiesch-Scholz, M.; Karst, M.** (Hannover)

Beeinflusst Knoblauch die Blutfliesseigenschaften und die Durchblutung bei progressiver systemischer Sklerose?: **Rapp, A.; Grohmann, G.; Oelzner, P.** (Jena); **Uehleke, B.** (Berlin); **Uhlemann, C.** (Jena)

Knochenmetastasen bei Mamma-Karzinom: **Teut, M.** (Berlin); **Warning, A.** (Essen)

Das anti-inflammatorische Potential von Padma 28 – Übersicht experimenteller Daten zur antiatherogenen Wirkung und Diskussion des Vielstoffkonzepts: **Überall, F.; Fuchs, D.** (Innsbruck); **Vennos, C.** (Schwerzenbach)

Aufbauen eines «Evidence House»: Herausforderungen und Lösungen für die komplementärmedizinische Forschung: **Jonas, W.B.** (Alexandria, VA)

Die Wirksamkeit von Balneotherapie bei chronischen Kreuzschmerzen – eine randomisierte, einfachblinde, kontrollierte Follow-up-Studie: **Balogh, Z.; Ördögh, J.; Gász, A.; Német, L.** (Kehidakustány); **Bender, T.** (Budapest)

Einflüsse geopathischer Störzonen auf den menschlichen Organismus: Nachweis stressender Effekte und Möglichkeit für Harmonisierung: **Hacker, G.W.; Pawlak, E.; Pauer, G.; Tichy, G.; Jell, H.; Posch, G.; Kraibacher, G.; Aigner, A.; Hutter, J.** (Salzburg)

Spontane ultraschwache Photonenenmission von biologischen Systemen und das endogene Lichtfeld: **Schwabl. H.** (Schwerzenbach); **Klima, H.** (Wien)

Weitere Informationen unter
www.karger.com/fok

- Pay-per-View und Volltext-Zugang für Abonnenten
- Vollständiges Inhaltsverzeichnis
- Wissenschaftlicher Beirat
- Frei zugängliche Abstracts und ausgewählte Artikel
- Online-Probeheft
- Einreichen von Arbeiten/Richtlinien für Autoren
- Abonnement
- Free Alert Service
- Online Library Recommendation

Forschende Komplementärmedizin
Research in Complementary Medicine
2007: Band 14 mit 6 Heften
Sprachen: Deutsch, Englisch
ISSN 1661–4119 (print)
ISSN 1661–4127 (online)

Aufgeführt in bibliographischen Diensten und *in Current Contents®*, MEDLINE.

Bestellformular

Ich kann diese Bestellung innerhalb zwei Wochen durch eine einfache Mitteilung an den Verlag widerrufen. Das Abonnement gilt zunächst für ein Jahr und verlängert sich um jeweils ein weiteres Jahr, wenn ich die Zeitschrift nicht bis 1. Dezember des laufenden Jahres abbestelle.

S. Karger
Verlag für Medizin und Naturwissenschaften GmbH
Lörracher Strasse 16A
D-79115 Freiburg (Deutschland)
Tel. +49 761 45 20 70
Fax +49 761 45 20 714
E-Mail: information@karger.de
www.karger.de

Ich abonniere
die Zeitschrift **Forschende Komplementärmedizin**
ab Jahrgang ________

☐ Print EUR 164.–
☐ Online EUR 164.–
☐ Print und Online kombiniert EUR 208.–

zum Sonderpreis für:
☐ Studenten/Ärzte in Weiterbildung
Mitglied einer Gesellschaft:
☐ DGEIM ☐ gamed ☐ GPhy
☐ Hufeland ☐ ISCMR ☐ Koop-Phyto
☐ SVHA ☐ Gesell. f. Arzneipflanzenforschung

☐ Print EUR 82.–
☐ Online EUR 82.–
☐ Print und Online kombiniert EUR 104.–

Diese Preise gelten für 2007 und verstehen sich inkl. MWSt., zzgl. EUR 18.– Versandkosten für Print-Abo.

☐ Bitte senden Sie mir ein kostenloses Probeheft von **Forschende Komplementärmedizin**

Ich bezahle
☐ mit Scheck ☐ auf Rechnung

Bitte belasten Sie diese Bestellung meiner Kreditkarte
☐ American Express ☐ MasterCard ☐ Visa

Karten-Nr: ________ Gültig bis: ________

Kartenprüfnummer (auf der Rückseite der Kreditkarte im Unterschriftenfeld): ________

Ich ermächtige die S. Karger GmbH bis auf Widerruf, jährlich meine Abonnement-Gebühren im Lastschriftverfahren abzubuchen (nur innerhalb Deutschlands möglich)

bei Bank oder Post: ________

in: ________ BLZ: ________

Giro-Konto-Nr: ________

Meine Postanschrift lautet (Blockschrift):

____

____

Tel.: ________ Datum/Unterschrift: ________

KF07034S

KARGER